PROMOTING PUBLIC MENTAL HEALTH AND WELL-BEING

Principles into Practice

Jean S. Brown, Alyson M. Learmonth and
Catherine J. Mackereth

Foreword by John R. Ashton

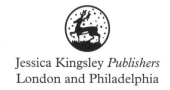

Jessica Kingsley *Publishers*
London and Philadelphia

First published in 2015
by Jessica Kingsley Publishers
73 Collier Street
London N1 9BE, UK
and
400 Market Street, Suite 400
Philadelphia, PA 19106, USA

www.jkp.com

Library of Congress Cataloging in Publication Data
Brown, Jean S., 1954- , author.
  Promoting public mental health and wellbeing / Jean S. Brown,
Alyson M. Learmonth, and Catherine J. Mackereth.
      p. ; cm.
  Includes bibliographical references and index.
  ISBN 978-1-84905-567-3 (alk. paper)
  I. Learmonth, Alyson M., author. II. Mackereth, Catherine J., author. III. Title.
  [DNLM: 1. Health Promotion. 2. Mental Health Services--
organization & administration. 3. Health Behavior. WM 30.1]
  RA776
  613--dc23

                    2014030708

British Library Cataloguing in Publication Data
A CIP catalogue record for this book is available from the British Library

ISBN 978 1 84905 567 3
eISBN 978 1 78450 004 7

Printed and bound in Great Britain by Bell and Bain Ltd, Glasgow

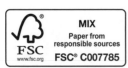

CONTENTS

Chapter 9 Extended case study: Improving mental health and well-being in people with long-term conditions 207

Conclusion A whole system for public mental health 232

FOREWORD

Once upon a time in the early 1960s, when every day was summer and the baby boomers believed that revolution was just around the corner, a psychiatrist by the name of Gerald Caplan published *An Approach to Community Mental Health* (Caplan 1961). What happened next?

For the past 50 years, Caplan's insights into public mental health have been eclipsed by a treatment model of mental health and illness, but finally the wheel is turning. The evidence is overwhelming that the burden of disease of mental ill health is vast and threatens not just our enjoyment of the fruits of 21st-century life and our pursuit of happiness, but the very viability and sustainability of health services themselves. A new paradigm is needed, based on the translation of New Public Health thinking into the mental health arena. It has been slow to come, but the steady stream of new texts is a sign that it is on its way.

This offering by Brown, Learmonth and Mackereth is a bold attempt to meet the need for a comprehensive but practical guide to the field. It builds on a life-cycle approach and the concepts of the Ottawa Charter to give commissioners and practitioners a ready diet for transforming both approaches and services. Importantly, it stresses the necessity to build on assets for mental health and resilience, rather than dwelling on deficits, and addresses the structural issues at a societal level that require political action. It will spawn a rich research agenda and will sit well on the shelf beside Gerald Caplan.

Professor John R. Ashton CBE MSc FFPH FRCP
FRCPsych, President, UK Faculty of Public Health

ACKNOWLEDGEMENTS

Many people have influenced us during our professional development, and we are grateful to all of them for their contributions. During the actual writing of this book the following have made time to read and give us their feedback from their diverse perspectives, which has been invaluable in shaping the final product: Edmund Derrick, Elaine Francis, Pauline Craig, Su Mably and Leslie Rudd. Thank you also to Peter Wright, Gary Carr and Paul Christer for their help with the table in the Conclusion. Any mistakes that remain are of course our own responsibility!

WHAT CREATES MENTAL HEALTH AND WELL-BEING?

What do we mean by mental health and well-being? Are you flourishing or languishing? Are you well or ill? What is the two-way relationship between decisions that affect your life chances and your mental state? What is our social responsibility for creating the optimum conditions for happiness? Who benefits? Why? Who decides? Are we taking account of the needs of future generations?

These are some of the questions we address in this book. This introduction sets out the scope of the book in relation to mental health, ill health and well-being, public health, health promotion and public mental health interventions. It goes on to explain its underlying values, to give a brief overview of the organization of the book and finally to identify who we hope will read it.

The aim of the book is to give a succinct introduction to the complex issue of mental health and well-being, drawing on evidence, in a way that is useful to a wide range of practitioners and decision-makers. The book also includes an extensive References section to assist readers to follow up any area on which they would like more detail.

WHAT ARE WE TALKING ABOUT?

Health can be defined in many ways. In 1948 the World Health Organization (WHO) set out the following: 'Health is a state of complete physical, mental and social wellbeing and not merely the absence of disease or infirmity' (WHO 1948, p.2). By 1984, this had been refined to define health as:

the extent to which an individual or a group is able to realise aspirations and satisfy needs, and to change or cope with the environment. Health is a resource for everyday life, not the objective of living; it is a positive concept, emphasizing social and personal resources as well as physical capabilities. (WHO 2009b, p.29)

It is clear that mental health and well-being are closely linked with generic concepts of health. The terms 'mental health', 'mental well-being' and 'emotional well-being' are often used interchangeably. 'Indeed "mental health" is often used instead of "mental illness"' (Mackereth 2009, p.9). Mental health, however, is a positive state, not just an absence of mental disease or illness.

Mental health is described by WHO as 'a state of wellbeing in which the individual realises his or her own abilities, can cope with the normal stresses of life, can work productively and fruitfully, and is able to make a contribution to his or her community' (WHO 2013, p.3).

Well-being has been defined as:

a dynamic state, in which the individual is able to develop their potential, work productively and creatively, build strong and positive relationships with others, and contribute to their community. It is enhanced when an individual is able to fulfil their personal and social goals and achieve a sense of purpose in society. (Foresight Mental Wellbeing and Capital Project 2008, p.10)

Although definitions of positive mental health vary, they generally include four elements: thinking; feeling; relationships; and meaning (Friedli 2009).

The relationship between mental health, illness and well-being can usefully be explored by thinking of two axes: a vertical line going from optimal well-being (flourishing) to minimal well-being (languishing); and a horizontal line going from high levels of mental illness to low levels of mental illness (The Scottish Government 2007). This creates four quadrants that may be helpful for considering various combinations. For example: someone can have a diagnosis of mental illness, and still be flourishing; or conversely someone can have no mental illness, but a very poor level of mental well-being (languishing). Mental health and well-being can therefore be considered at all stages of life, and despite a diagnosis of mental illness. We have adopted this position in compiling our material for this book.

Because learning disability presents its own unique issues, we have not attempted to address it here, except when discussing the fact that people with learning disabilities are more vulnerable to poor well-being or mental illness. Of course people with learning disabilities can also flourish or languish. We have also chosen not to discuss mental illness arising from organic disease, such as dementia or syphilis. A further issue that we do not address is the genetic component of mental illness, as the focus of the book is on public mental health and well-being, rather than illness, and the genetic component is an area upon which public health interventions are unlikely to have a direct impact.

Traditionally, public health has considered three overlapping aspects of disease prevention:

1. Primary prevention targets whole populations and involves community and personal action that reduces the chances of ill health. It addresses the social determinants of poor health as well as lifestyle and is sometimes referred to as 'upstream'.

2. Secondary prevention targets those vulnerable to disease and involves engaging this group in an appropriate lifestyle, and early detection of illness in order to prevent its progression.

3. Tertiary prevention involves working with people with established ill health to promote recovery and prevent (or reduce the risk of) recurrence.

Prevention interventions may relate to a range of associated issues, including those related to determinants of health, such as: deprivation and inequalities; promoting good physical health through lifestyle measures; and reducing high-risk behaviour such as violence and abuse. Overall, the goal is to reduce levels of mental disorder.

Early intervention occurs in the following areas: early diagnosis and treatment of mental disorder; promotion of physical health and prevention of health risk behaviour in those developing mental disorder; and the promotion of recovery through early provision of a range of interventions. The goal is to reduce the harm arising from the mental disorder.

Treatment and rehabilitation aim to promote recovery and prevent the risk of recurrence. Tackling stigma and discrimination is important to prevention at all three levels. Chapter 1 scopes the most common mental disorders in terms of the scale of the problem. In this book the focus is on prevention and early intervention, and to some extent rehabilitation. Clinical issues of treatment or therapy are not addressed, although documenting the way that the wider determinants affect mental health and well-being should be of value to those working in these fields.

The promotion of health, which aims to improve quality of life, can also occur at three levels, reflecting the three levels of prevention described above: primary (the whole population); secondary (targeted to groups at high risk); and tertiary (working with groups who have established illness to treat or prevent recurrence).

Mental health promotion interventions focus on increasing mental health and well-being. One framework for this follows a life course sequence, and this is expanded on in Chapter 4. The settings approach is another way of designing interventions and is discussed in Chapter 6.

Public mental health interventions result in:

- economic savings by reducing the costs of mental disorder through prevention and improved outcomes as a result of early intervention
- economic savings associated with improved well-being, such as reduced welfare dependency, reduced use of health and social care services, less crime and greater social cohesion
- economic savings resulting from reduced health risk behaviour and subsequent physical illness
- economic benefits associated with improved well-being as a consequence of improved educational outcomes, higher employment rates and greater economic productivity.

Mental health and well-being is fundamental to public health and health improvement. Good mental health provides the bedrock for good physical health and for a range of other important life skills, capacities and capabilities (JCPMH 2013).

UNDERLYING PRINCIPLES

There are four key principles informing this book, which are used to underpin the concluding section in each chapter to demonstrate how principles have been translated into practice. The four principles are the following:

- Mental health and well-being is a holistic concept, not just focusing on illness, and is central to an individual's social purpose, autonomy and ability to make life choices.

- Social, economic, political, cultural and environmental factors, the 'determinants of health', must be addressed if we are to enhance mental health and well-being.

- Two key public health tools that should be consistently applied are the assessment of health care need in the population concerned and the use of systematically assessed evidence about what works.

- Community engagement is central to public mental health and is concerned with involving communities, users and carers in helping to frame appropriate priorities, and build on existing assets.

We place a high value on 'enabling people to increase control over, and to improve, their health' (WHO 1986, p.1). The 'healthy society' is one in which people are empowered as individuals and where the emphasis in public policy is on meeting needs, equalizing opportunities and enhancing social justice.

The theoretical underpinnings for this stance have been most thoroughly developed by Seedhouse (1988). He developed an 'ethical grid' to assist health practitioners to reflect systematically on situations and take ethically informed decisions.[1] He emphasizes that there is rarely a 'correct' answer, but the issue of enhancing autonomy is central to everyone who intends to create better health.

The book also includes, where it is relevant to mental health and well-being, an intergenerational perspective on inequality, putting future generations' moral claims on to the agenda. This builds on the arguments developed by Graham (2010, 2012) that we are currently borrowing environmental capital from future generations with no intention or ability to repay it.

In order to create a framework for the book, we have made use of the Ottawa Charter for Health Promotion, which identified the following five essential areas for action underlying a strategy to fundamentally change health and well-being:

---

1   Seedhouse's ethical grid involves potential consideration from four key perspectives: Does the proposed action further equity, respect and autonomy? What are your duties and motives? Will the consequences of the action be good, and if so for whom? How does the action weigh up against external criteria such as legal considerations, evidence of effectiveness or legal responsibilities?

- Build healthy public policy.
- Strengthen community action.
- Develop personal skills.
- Create supportive environments.
- Reorientate services.

(WHO 1986)

Each of these is explained further in Chapters 5 and 6.

The Ottawa Charter also identified prerequisites for health, an essential foundation for improvements in health to occur: 'The fundamental conditions and resources for health are peace, shelter, education, food, income, a stable eco-system, sustainable resources, social justice and equity' (*ibid.*, p.1).

WHO and its Regional Offices have updated this early strategy a number of times. The most recent European example is *Health 2020: A European Policy Framework Across Government and Society for Health and Wellbeing*, which recognizes that real improvements in health can only result from working to improve health for all at the same time as reducing inequalities. A linked strategic objective is to improve leadership and participatory governance related to health (WHO Regional Office for Europe 2012).

The strategy sets out four key priority areas for working together. The first is empowerment of people and investing in health through a life course approach, followed by tackling Europe's major health challenges. The third is to strengthen people-centred health systems and capacity in all aspects of public health. The final priority is to create supportive environments and resilient communities. Working together includes a combination of individuals and collective efforts involving civil society and the business sector, within and among European Member States, to address these priorities.

So, over the last 25 years, high-level strategic thinking has consistently indicated that we need to work with whole systems if we are to effectively improve health. We have chosen to apply the original five headings from the Ottawa Charter to mental health and well-being to underpin our strategic thinking, the translation of that strategic thinking into operational plans and the illustrative case studies. We chose them rather than some of the later developments arising from this seminal work because of their holistic nature, embracing: the role of personal responsibility and action at a community level; the need to reorientate health services; the importance of a supportive environment to create health; and the impact of public policy at a global and national level. We have, however, interpreted the reorientation of health services to include integrated health and social care, where appropriate. We believe also that the five Ottawa Charter headings provide a framework that is easy to understand.

ORGANIZATION OF THE MATERIAL

In tackling this complex subject, we have adopted the following sequence.

Chapter 1 gives an overview of mental health policy and the scale of the problem and includes a discussion of outcomes and ways to measure population well-being.

Chapter 2 explores the two-way relationship between social, economic and environmental circumstances, and mental health and well-being. It includes all of the prerequisites for health mentioned in the Ottawa Charter and listed earlier, although shelter is included both here (housing) and in the next chapter (homelessness), and food is covered both here and in Chapter 4.

Chapters 3 and 4 consider the personal circumstances that make people more resilient or vulnerable to poor mental health (life stage, being part of a marginalized group, living circumstances, health-related behaviour).

Chapter 5 discusses what we know about the development of strategies that improve health, in particular mental health and well-being; and Chapter 6 describes some ways to translate these strategies into operational delivery by organizations and practitioners. Both of these two chapters explain and use the Ottawa Charter's five areas for action as headings: building healthy public policy, strengthening community action, building personal skills, creating a supportive environment, and reorientating health care services. Chapter 6 includes evidence-based interventions, with further examples in each of the extended case studies.

Chapters 7, 8 and 9 are three extended case studies where the ideas presented in the earlier chapters are applied to examples of situations with very different characteristics: a specific social problem (suicide);

a population group (young Black and Minority Ethnic groups); and a medically defined problem (people with long-term conditions). The following criteria have been used in each of these chapters, and each is fully explained in the first six chapters as indicated in brackets against each bullet point. The sequence has been chosen to take the reader through the logical steps of a public health analysis, in relation to each case study:

- Groups in the population who are affected (drawing mainly from chapters 3 and 4).
- Wider determinants of health (drawing mainly from chapter 2).
- Evidence base, effectiveness and cost effectiveness of interventions (drawing on Chapters 2, 3, 4, 5 and 6):
  - building healthy public policy
  - strengthening community action
  - building personal skills
  - creating supportive environments
  - reorientating health care services.
- Quality assurance, health equity audit and evaluation (drawing on Chapters 1, 5 and 6).

WHO IS IT FOR?

Our goal in writing this book has been to make public health thinking about mental health and well-being accessible to people who 'need to know' across the UK. With this accessibility in mind, we have tried to avoid jargon wherever possible: where technical language is unavoidable, we have provided explanations. In particular, we have been thinking of:

- agencies involved in high-level strategic thinking about mental health and well-being at a population level, such as health and social care commissioners and providers, the voluntary sector, and other parts of the public sector, for example maternity and children's services, housing, leisure, regulatory services, criminal justice, education, and cultural services including libraries, galleries and museums
- front-line service providers in all these fields

- post-graduate students in the wide range of disciplines leading to front-line provision or strategy development related to mental health and well-being, such as commissioning, mental health nursing, primary care, psychology, psychiatry, therapy, public health, pastoral care, social work, health visiting, school nursing, teaching, health sciences, spatial planning, environmental health, trading standards and housing.

We have avoided comparative information about the specific health care systems of the four UK nations, on the grounds that it is complex information available elsewhere, and that health care services are not the primary focus of this book. However, the group identified in the first of the three points above, agencies involved in high-level strategic thinking about mental health and well-being at a population level, matches so closely with English Health and Wellbeing Boards[2] that it is worth commenting briefly on them. These were established in 2013, as part of the new responsibility given to Local Authorities for Health and Well-being under the Health and Social Care Act 2012. The Health and Wellbeing Boards have a statutory responsibility to produce two particular related documents: a Joint Strategic Needs Assessment (JSNA) and a Joint Health and Wellbeing Strategy (JHWS). Together, these are intended to improve the health and well-being of the local community and reduce inequalities for all ages (DH 2013g).

---

2   The Health and Social Care Act 2012 prescribes a core statutory membership of at least one elected representative, nominated by either the leader of the council, the mayor or in some cases by the local authority, a representative from each Clinical Commissioning Group (CCG) (see below) whose area falls within, or coincides with, the local authority area, the local authority directors of adult social services, children's services and public health, and a representative from the local Healthwatch organization. In some places they may also include representatives from service providers, fire and rescue services, universities, military populations, criminal justice agencies and local voluntary and community sector organizations. An important part of the role of Health and Wellbeing Boards is to shape local health and care services, deciding how they will be bought and delivered. Central to their success is the focus on health and care services working together (DH n.d. a).

Clinical Commissioning Groups (CCGs) are clinically led groups that include all of the GP groups in their geographical area. They are overseen by NHS England. CCGs operate by commissioning (or buying) health care services, including mental health services. They work with patients and health care professionals and in partnership with local communities and local authorities. On their governing body, CCGs have, in addition to GPs, at least one registered nurse and a doctor who is a secondary care specialist. Their boundaries are normally coterminous with those of local authorities (RCN 2013).

While the responsibility for 'Health and Well-being' is not statutory in other parts of the UK, similar players are involved. For example, Scotland's Public Bodies (Joint Working) (Scotland) Bill 2013 stresses the use of integrated budgets and joint accountability across health and social care. In addition all Community Planning Partnerships should have a focus on the following key priorities where the aim should be to achieve transformational, not incremental, performance improvement: economic recovery and growth; employment; early years; safer and stronger communities, and reducing offending; health inequalities and physical activity; and outcomes for older people (The Scottish Government and COSLA 2012). The potential to improve not just physical health but mental health and well-being is widely recognized.

It is the hope of the authors that this 'primer' gives a useful overview of this complex subject in a way that you the reader can quickly find the material you need. In this way, it may make its own contribution to developing both strategy and practice in an area of work that is vital in its own right, and has significant implications for other aspects of health inequalities.

Chapter 1

MEASURING OUTCOMES RELATED TO MENTAL HEALTH AND WELL-BEING

WHAT DO WE WANT TO ACHIEVE?

KEY POINTS

- The policy context across the four parts of the UK is similar in relation to improved outcomes for people with mental health problems.

- In 2012/2013, 6 per cent of adults aged over 18 (2.6 million people in England) were on practice depression registers.

- A household survey suggested that more than 16 per cent of adults in England met the diagnostic criteria for at least one common mental disorder.

- Investing in the promotion of well-being, prevention of mental disorder and early treatment of mental disorder results in significant economic savings, even in the short term.

- Mental health and well-being features in all of the outcomes frameworks set out for the NHS, public health, social care and primary care.

- Measuring mental health and well-being at a population level is a developing field.

INTRODUCTION

An overarching goal of achieving good mental health and well-being for the whole population has recently become an explicit part of UK government policy. However, like any political action, it cannot be left as a dream. This leads to debate: What goals are realistic? How can progress towards them be measured? This chapter gives a brief overview of the current landscape of mental health and well-being from this perspective. Quite often we find that what we want to measure cannot be directly measured, so we may have to use 'proxy measures' – measures of something that is related in some way – instead. Examples include estimating need by the number of people already accessing certain services. Before discussing such examples, this chapter considers the desired outcomes that are laid out in various UK mental health policies and strategies.

TARGETS IN MENTAL HEALTH POLICIES

Key points from national policies and strategies are shown below. In general, the policies refer to *improving* mental health and well-being. Since they are designed specifically for mental health, they also have a focus on services for those with mental health problems, talking of aspects such as early identification and treatment of problems, user–carer involvement, equality of service provision and multi-agency collaboration. Reducing service costs is often a desired outcome. Overall there may be a large variety of targets and many elements that need to be measured to track any progress towards those targets.

National mental health policies
No Health without Mental Health: A Cross-government Mental Health Outcomes Strategy for People of All Ages. (England (HM Government and DH 2011))

This mental health outcomes strategy looks to communities, as well as the state, to promote independence and choice, reflecting the recent vision for adult social care. It sets out how the government, working with all sectors of the community and taking a life course approach, will:

- Improve the mental health and well-being of the population and keep people well.
- Improve outcomes for people with mental health problems through high-quality services that are equally accessible to all.

The six broad objectives are as follows:

- More people will have good mental health.
- More people with mental health problems will recover.
- More people with mental health problems will have good physical health.
- More people will have a positive experience of care and support.
- Fewer people will suffer avoidable harm.
- Fewer people will experience stigma and discrimination.

Together for Mental Health: A Strategy for Mental Health and Wellbeing in Wales (Wales (Welsh Government 2012))

This is a ten-year strategy for improving the lives of people using mental health services, their carers and their families. At the heart of the strategy is the Mental Health (Wales) Measure 2010, which places legal duties on health boards and local authorities to improve support for people with mental ill health.

The strategy has six high-level outcomes:

- The mental health and well-being of the whole population is improved.
- The impact of mental health problems and/or mental illness on individuals of all ages, their families and carers, communities and the economy more widely is better recognized and reduced.
- Inequalities, stigma and discrimination suffered by people experiencing mental health problems and mental illness are reduced.
- Individuals have a better experience of the support and treatment they receive and have an increased feeling of input and control over related decisions.
- Access to, and the quality of, preventative measures, early intervention and treatment services are improved and more people recover as a result.

- The values, attitudes and skills of those treating or supporting individuals of all ages with mental health problems or mental illness are improved.

Mental Health Strategy for Scotland 2012–2015 (Scotland (The Scottish Government 2012d))

This has the vision that by 2020 everyone is able to live longer, healthier lives at home, or in a homely setting. The strategy focuses on a range of improvements and interventions that are in accordance with the best evidence for return against investment over time, including:

- Early intervention for conduct disorder in children through evidence-based parenting programmes.
- Treating depression in those with long-term conditions such as diabetes.
- Early diagnosis and treatment of depression.
- Eearly detection and treatment of psychosis.

Its seven themes for mental health are:

- Working more effectively with families and carers.
- Embedding more peer-to-peer work and support.
- Increasing the support for self-management and self-help approaches.
- Extending the anti-stigma agenda forward to include further work on discrimination.
- Focusing on the rights of those with mental illness.
- Developing the outcomes approach to include personal, social and clinical outcomes.
- Ensuring that we use new technology effectively as a mechanism for providing information and delivering evidence-based services.

Service Framework for Mental Health and Wellbeing (Northern Ireland (DHSS&PS 2011))

This framework aims to improve the mental health and well-being of the population of Northern Ireland, reduce inequalities and improve the quality of health and social care in relation to mental health.

The framework includes 58 standards, some appropriate to specific groups, such as young people or the homeless. Key messages are that the services should:

- be high quality
- allow equitable access to all groups
- provide appropriate integrated, multi-agency support
- involve prevention as well as treatment
- involve users and carers in the planning, development and monitoring of mental health services.

We have limited our discussion in this section to 'mental health policy'. As we shall see later, this is only a tiny fraction of the policy that can have an effect on mental health and well-being. Throughout subsequent chapters we refer to other policies and strategies that are extremely relevant to mental well-being and particularly the prevention of mental ill health and the enhancement of general well-being. In the next few sections of this chapter, we shall look at some of the possible targets related to mental well-being and the issues around measuring progress.

MEASURING NUMBERS OF PEOPLE WITH PARTICULAR MENTAL HEALTH CONDITIONS

Although it is a measure of problems rather than wellness, it can be useful to have an idea of how many people are suffering from mental health conditions. These prevalence figures are valuable particularly to service planners, to help them estimate the demand for services such as inpatient beds or community psychiatric nurses. An estimated one in four people will suffer from a mental health problem over the course of a year (Mental Health Foundation n.d. b).

There are many types of mental disorder, including the following (definitions from NHSIC 2009):

- Psychotic disorders 'produce disturbances in thinking and perception severe enough to distort perception of reality. The main types are schizophrenia and affective psychosis, such as bipolar disorder' (p.89).

- Antisocial and borderline personality disorders are 'longstanding, ingrained distortions of personality that interfere with the ability to make and sustain relationships' (p.105).

- Common mental disorders – also known as neurotic disorders – are 'mental conditions that cause marked emotional distress and interfere with daily function but do not usually affect insight and cognition' (p.25). The term covers depression and anxiety (including phobias, panic disorders and obsessive compulsive disorder).

Other conditions include post-traumatic stress disorder (PTSD), attention deficit hyperactivity disorder (ADHD), eating disorders, alcohol and drug dependence and gambling dependence.

GP practice information can help to provide estimates of how widespread some conditions are. In 2012/2013, in England, of those who were registered with GP practices, 0.8 per cent were on practice registers of people with schizophrenia, bipolar affective disorder and other psychoses, and 6 per cent of adults aged more than 18 (2.6 million people) were on practice depression registers (HSCIC 2013a). These figures are likely to be underestimates of the scale of the problem, partly because GP practices do not have to provide the information (see the section below on quality outcomes frameworks), partly because of non-reporting from those registered with a GP and partly because not everyone is registered with a GP (and, as we shall see later, some of the most vulnerable people are those who may not be registered, such as the homeless).

Sometimes the only available data are estimates from surveys, one of the most commonly used of which, the Adult Psychiatric Morbidity Survey (NHSIC 2009), has suggested that more than 16 per cent of adults met the diagnostic criteria for at least one common mental disorder in the week prior to interview.

To a large extent, our focus will be on those conditions that are preventable, particularly the common mental disorder, depression. As described in Chapter 6, there are many actions that can be taken to help reduce the likelihood of suffering from depression.

MEASURING SERVICE UPTAKE

Some items are routinely measured to show progress in terms of service uptake. Examples include:

- numbers of patients receiving psychological therapies
- numbers of patients admitted to hospital for particular mental health conditions, which can normally be calculated fairly easily from hospital episode statistics but is complicated when patients have more than one condition
- the number of people receiving specialist mental health care outside of the hospital setting
- numbers of prescriptions given for particular mental health problems, which can be obtained but is complicated because some drugs are used to treat a variety of both physical and mental health problems.

Although these do not tell us how many people have good mental health or well-being, they allow us to see how many are taking up services because they are in need of improving their mental health. Even this will not be a complete picture of the numbers actually needing services – there may be others who would benefit from help but are not accessing it, from choice or because of stigma, or because of a limited availability of services. If it is the latter, there may well be statistics to show how many people are on a waiting list for particular services.

Figures like these will contribute to a picture of how things are changing over time, but changes may not be a consequence of changes in a population's mental health, but to a range of other factors, such as:

- improvements in diagnostic techniques (so that there seems to be a sudden jump in the number with a particular condition, whereas really it is just that more have been diagnosed)
- changes in availability of services – an increase in the number of clinics may allow larger numbers of patients to receive treatment over a certain time period
- changes in diagnostic classifications so that comparison over time is not possible – for example, a condition being split into sub-classifications or moved into a different category in the *Diagnostic and Statistical Manual of Mental Disorders* (DSM) (American Psychiatric Association 2013a)

- improvements or changes in the delivery of treatment – if treatment becomes available that can be delivered at home (in the community) rather than the patient having to visit a hospital clinic, this would show up as a decrease in the numbers accessing hospital services but an increase in community activity.

MEASURING CHANGE IN SERVICE PERSONNEL

The number of staff involved in delivering services may be used to assess the need or potential for change. Examples of data routinely recorded may include:

- numbers of staff delivering specialist mental health services in hospital
- numbers of staff delivering community mental health services.

Again, while this does not tell us how many people have good or poor mental well-being, it helps to present the picture of the services provided. New staffing guidance emerged in 2013 in England to help decision-makers to make the right decisions about nursing care staffing and capability (NHS England 2013).

MEASURING SUCCESS OF SERVICES

It is not always possible to say that a mental health condition has been 'cured'. Some mental health conditions, particularly depression, are akin to long-term physical health problems, which will not go away but can be addressed to improve the patient's ability to live a 'normal' life, or treated in order to minimize discomfort. There are measures that can indicate that there has been some success with treatment, including:

- average length of stay in hospital for mental health conditions – in general, patients and families prefer short hospital stays, if they are necessary at all (Horvitz-Lennon *et al.* 2001), and from the health service's viewpoint, hospital stays prove very expensive
- readmissions to hospital within a certain period after discharge – when patients have been discharged following a stay for a mental health condition but then have to be readmitted for the same condition, it can be because the discharge happened too early and the patient was not really ready for discharge.

There are also individual measures of progress as assessed by patients (discussed later in this chapter), which can help to provide an overall picture of service success.

Different ways that services can evaluate their delivery will be outlined in Chapters 5 and 6. One example is social return on investment (SROI), developed to evaluate the social, economic and environmental value of activities and interventions. It is concerned with tackling inequalities, as well as improving well-being (Nicholls *et al.* 2012). This approach attaches financial values to social, environmental and economic outcomes, enabling comparisons to be made: for example, it may be found that £1 invested will deliver £2 of social value.

FINANCIAL MEASUREMENT AND THE FINANCIAL IMPERATIVE

Even if we cannot always get accurate assessments of the numbers of people who need help for mental health conditions, one area where information is available is that of expenditure on services. For mental health, the cost of services is very high, so it can easily become a target area for spending cuts.

Poor mental health has a huge impact, not just on the individual, but also on the national economy: the total cost of poor mental health problems is estimated at nearly £26 billion per annum, with employees taking, on average, seven days off work a year for health reasons, some 40 per cent as a consequence of mental health problems (Glasgow Centre for Population Health 2011; Sainsbury Centre for Mental Health 2007). The financial costs of loss of productivity related to poor mental health extends beyond the losses associated with sickness absence, to include 'presenteeism', wherein people continue to attend work, despite functioning at a less than optimum capacity (Friedli 2009). The costs are estimated at £1.5 billion a year in reduced productivity (SCMH 2007).

There are additional issues around caring. There are some five million people looking after an ill, disabled or frail family member, friend or partner without being paid. Provision of this care would cost social services and the NHS an estimated £119 billion per year – compared to the total cost of the NHS at £98.8 billion in the financial year 2009/2010 (Buckner and Yeandle 2011).

Investment in the promotion of mental well-being, prevention of mental disorder and early treatment of mental disorder results in significant economic savings even in the short term. As a consequence of the broad impact of mental disorder and well-being, these savings occur in health, social care, criminal justice and other public sectors. For example, for every £1 invested in public mental health interventions, net savings are £44 from 'suicide prevention through GP training' and £84 from 'school-based social and emotional learning programmes' (JCPMH 2013, p.11).

OUTCOMES FRAMEWORKS

The last decade has seen the development of several 'outcomes frameworks'. These lay out desired outcomes (often identified to relate to government policy) for specific services. We shall look briefly at some of the national outcomes frameworks. Outcomes are effectively the results of interventions – changes that have been brought about by an activity or action. They can be difficult to measure (for example, how much better someone is feeling). They differ from outputs, which are usually easier to measure and can provide information such as how many activities have taken place (for example, the number of people who have undergone therapy).

Outcomes frameworks for statutory services

In England there are three complementary outcomes frameworks:

- The NHS Outcomes Framework 2014–2015 (DH 2013f) sets out the outcomes and corresponding indicators that will be used to hold NHS England to account for improvements in health outcomes.
- The Public Health Outcomes Framework (DH 2012b) supports the whole public health system (nationally and locally).
- The Adult Social Care Outcomes Framework (DH 2012a) is used both locally and nationally in England to set priorities for care and support, measure progress and strengthen transparency and accountability.

Scotland's Community Care Outcomes Framework (The Scottish Government 2012c) aims to improve joint delivery of community care services; its National Outcomes describe what the government wants to achieve over the next ten years; and its Health Improvement, Efficiency, Access and Appropriate Treatment (HEAT) targets contribute towards the delivery of its Purpose and National Outcomes (The Scottish Government 2012b). Wales is developing an NHS Outcomes Framework (Welsh Government 2014) in line with the commitment in Together for Health, and Northern Ireland is implementing the findings of a consultation on transforming its Health and Social Care services (DHSS&PS 2014).

The following are some of the outcomes directly applicable to mental health and occurring in at least one of the frameworks (and frequently in several):

- reducing numbers of people dying prematurely:
    - in people with serious mental illness
    - suicide
- health improvement:
    - hospital admissions caused by unintentional and deliberate injuries in under 18s
    - emotional well-being of looked-after children (not yet finalized)
    - improving outcomes from planned treatments – total health gain as assessed by patients for psychological therapies
    - increase the average score of adults on the Warwick-Edinburgh Mental Well-Being Scale (WEMWBS)
- enhancing quality of life for people with mental illness
- ensuring that people have a positive experience of care:
    - people, including those involved in making decisions on social care, respect the dignity of the individual and ensure support is sensitive to the circumstances of each individual
    - improving experience of health care for people with mental illness – patient experience of community mental health services
    - percentage of users and carers who are satisfied with their involvement in the design of care package

- ◦ faster access to specialist child and mental health services
- ◦ faster access to psychological therapies
- improving the wider determinants of health:
  - ◦ people with mental illness or disability in settled accommodation
  - ◦ percentage of community care service users feeling safe
  - ◦ people are able to find employment when they want, maintain a family and social life, contribute to community life and avoid loneliness or isolation
  - ◦ proportion of adults in contact with secondary mental health services in paid employment
  - ◦ proportion of adults in contact with secondary mental health services living independently, with or without support.

The Quality Outcomes Framework for General Practices

The Quality Outcomes Framework (DHSS&PS n.d.; HSCIC n.d. b; ISD Scotland n.d.; Welsh Government 2013b) is a voluntary incentive scheme for GP practices in the UK, rewarding them for how well they care for patients. It contains groups of indicators, against which practices score points according to their level of achievement. Examples include:

- monitoring:
  - ◦ whether the practice has a register of patients with particular mental health conditions
  - ◦ the proportions of those patients for whom records are kept of blood pressure, alcohol consumption or body mass index (BMI)

  (Although these are measuring record-keeping, rather than evidence of an improvement in health, they indicate that monitoring is being undertaken, which should improve outcomes for the patients.)
- patient and carer involvement:
  - ◦ the percentages of patients on the register who have a comprehensive care plan documented in the records agreed between individuals, their family and/or carers as appropriate

(Again this measures record-keeping but indicates that a process of user and carer involvement is established.)

- case-finding and assessment of depression. It is recommended that patients with certain long-term conditions are assessed for depression
  - the indicator used to record this 'case-finding' is the number of patients who have been assessed as a proportion of patients on the practice's related long-term conditions registers
  - in those patients with a new diagnosis of depression, this is the percentage of patients who have had an assessment of severity at the time of diagnosis

(Once again, it is process that is measured, but when patients are assessed in this way it should lead to early treatment.)

MEASURING WELL-BEING

Finding suitable outcome measures for a population's mental health and well-being is not straightforward and is frequently controversial. If the outcome is to improve general mental health and well-being, what is actually being measured? How can we find a measurement that will show that general mental health and well-being is improving?

Suicide rates

For some years, one measure that has repeatedly been used is that of suicide rates. This assumes that the rates of suicide in a population are an indication of that population's mental health, and that if rates are decreasing then the population's mental health is improving. These assumptions have been challenged for several reasons: suicide is only one tiny part of mental health problems, at the extreme end of a spectrum; the numbers of suicides are comparatively small, so that small rises or falls can quite dramatically affect rates; just because we can count the numbers of suicides does not mean that this is a good measure; and it may be one part of measuring mental illness but it does not measure mental well-being. Nonetheless, in spite of criticisms, it is used as a measure in many policies.

Well-being estimates

Many of the outcome measures already described are objective measures, but well-being is very much subjective – people will not all necessarily view well-being in the same way and, even with some kind of scoring system, may rank certain aspects of their lives and feelings very differently from one another. Approaches involving scoring are an established part of individual mental health assessment, measuring changes in a patient's feelings of well-being. Over the past few years there has been increasing use of these measurements at a population level, aggregating the scores to provide an estimate of a whole population's well-being. The following are brief descriptions of some of the most commonly used approaches.

The Warwick-Edinburgh Mental Well-being Scale (WEMWBS)

WEMWBS, along with its shorter version, the Short Warwick-Edinburgh Mental Well-Being Scale (SWEMWBS), is now a well-established system of measuring an individual's well-being. It is now routinely used in national surveys, including the Scottish Health Survey 2012 (The Scottish Government 2013), the Health Survey for Northern Ireland 2011/12 (DHSS&PS 2012a) and the Health Survey for England 2012 (ONS 2013c). Scotland uses the average score of adults on WEMWBS as its national indicator of mental well-being.

WEMWBS asks people to consider 14 statements, covering several aspects of life and living, such as: feelings of optimism and cheerfulness; being relaxed; satisfying interpersonal relationships; good levels of energy; feeling confident; and thinking clearly. Statements are positively worded (for example, 'I've been feeling optimistic…') and are given scores of 1 to 5, indicating how often people have felt a certain way, with 1 being 'none of the time' and 5 being 'all of the time'. The national surveys make use of mean scores.

The General Health Questionnaire (GHQ12)

GHQ12, also used in the National Health Surveys, is a measure of psychosocial health, consisting of 12 questions on concentration abilities, sleeping patterns, self-esteem, stress, despair, depression and confidence in the previous few weeks. A 4-point scale is used, and a score of 0 is given for a symptom being present 'not at all' or 'no more than usual', with a score of 1 given whenever the response is 'rather more than usual' or 'much more than usual'. Average scores out of 12 are used as a reflection of population psychosocial health.

Life satisfaction question

The Scottish Health Survey (The Scottish Government 2013) also uses a life satisfaction question. Life satisfaction is measured by asking participants to rate, on a scale of 0 to 10, how satisfied they are with their life in general (0 being 'extremely dissatisfied' and 10 'extremely satisfied'). Overall patterns of scores in the population are used to estimate proportions of people with the highest levels of satisfaction, people with average satisfaction levels and people with below average scores.

Short Form 36 health survey (SF-36)

The SF-36 contains questions about whether emotional problems (such as feeling depressed or anxious) have affected work or daily activities or interfered with normal social activities. Some of its questions assess general mood, with people indicating how much of the time recently they have felt full of energy, or been nervous or felt low or peaceful. It has been used, for example, in the Welsh Health Survey 2012 (Welsh Government 2013a), which reported a summary score for adults who reported currently being treated for mental illnesses.

ONS (Office for National Statistics) well-being questions

ONS uses a set of four questions to monitor personal well-being in the UK:

1. Overall, how satisfied are you with your life nowadays?
2. Overall, to what extent do you feel the things you do in your life are worthwhile?
3. Overall, how happy did you feel yesterday?
4. Overall, how anxious did you feel yesterday?

(ONS 2013e, p.2)

People are asked to give answers on a scale of 1 to 10, with 0 meaning 'not at all' and 10 meaning 'completely'. Although it is a snapshot, with people's feelings regarding 'yesterday' not necessarily being typical, it is hoped that overall, with a large sample of people responding, it will still enable a picture of changes over time to emerge. Results are presented either as averages or as proportions of people rating each aspect at the highest or lowest level.

Social trust question

The New Economics Foundation (NEF) (NEF 2012), in its recommendations to voluntary organizations and community groups delivering projects and services, suggests that they measure well-being using several approaches: SWEMWBS and the ONS subjective well-being questions described above, and a question on social trust, which is known to be a key factor for well-being. The social trust question (*ibid.*, p.11) is: 'Generally speaking, would you say that most people can be trusted, or that you can't be too careful in dealing with people?' Respondents give a score of 0 to 10, where 0 means you cannot be too careful and 10 means that most people can be trusted.

Clinician Reported Outcome Measures (also called Clinician Led Outcome Measures)

These are ways of measuring the outcomes of treatment as assessed by clinicians. One with widespread use in the UK is the Health of the Nation Outcome Scales (HoNOS), which considers 12 dimensions, which the clinician rates on a 5-point scale.

Patient reported measures

One aspect of patient reported measures is that of patient experience. Patient Reported Experience Measures (PREMs) have in recent years become one way of assessing how patients feel about the services they received. One specifically designed for mental health patients is the Community Mental Health Survey (Care Quality Commission 2013). Primarily designed for mental health trusts in England, to help them to improve their services, there are questions within it about people's medication and treatment, including how helpful recipients found some treatments to be, and views on the staff treating them. There are also questions on day-to-day living and the levels of support needed or provided.

There is currently much work going on to assess the outcomes of treatment and levels of care of patients, using patients' evaluations rather than clinicians' evaluations of progress. Some Patient Reported

Outcome Measures (PROMs) have been successfully collected and used for patients following treatment for procedures for various physical conditions, and this may be extended to cover some mental health conditions. Measures that are already used for general health (with elements relevant to mental well-being) include EuroQol's 'Quality of Life – 5 Dimensions' and 'Visual Analogue Scale', which measure quality of life, with patients rating five areas of life: mobility, self-care, usual activities, pain/discomfort and anxiety/depression.

There are several tools that help people to measure their own progress with the help of professionals. For example, the Recovery Star has the ten points of a star representing different dimensions of life, including daily living activities and not only mental or emotional health (Mental Health Foundation n.d. c). Users and helpers assess where the user is with regards to each dimension. When the exercise is repeated, perhaps months later, the user can see the progress being made.

FINDING APPROPRIATE INFORMATION

Surveys

Apart from the health surveys of each of the UK nations, other national surveys (for example, the Psychiatric Morbidity Survey (NHSIC 2009) mentioned earlier) can provide helpful health-based information. Local surveys can also be specifically designed with particular groups of patients or conditions in mind, but they tend to be very costly and time-consuming and can be inapplicable to a wider group.

Looking more widely, relevant information can also be obtained from surveys not specific to health, such as housing surveys or crime surveys, which can help to determine whether the factors affecting mental health are changing or are significantly different in certain areas.

Dashboards and profiles

A range of profiles is produced by certain national agencies, some focusing largely on physical health but with elements very relevant to mental well-being. Profiles use a variety of sources, which can sometimes suggest other potential routes of investigation. Although they may present only a limited set of facts, they can be valuable for comparing districts, as well as looking at change over time. An example is the Community Mental Health Profile (NEPHO 2013), which presents a range of mental health information for local authorities in England, including risk factors, prevalence of conditions and service information. Another example is the Scottish Government's profile of Child and Adolescent Mental Health (The Scottish Government 2012a), assessing progress towards the Mental Health Strategy for Scotland.

A dashboard is a type of profile, usually used to highlight issues or to show progress against objectives in a policy. One example is England's first annual mental health dashboard (DH 2013e), which uses publicly available information and aims to show progress against the objectives of its *No Health without Mental Health* strategy.

Government statistics

As well as publishing the health surveys and information from the quality outcomes frameworks mentioned above, each of the four nations publishes information on its services that can help to identify need or demand. Some routine hospital episode statistics, based on certain details of every hospital stay, are publicly available at a national level and arrangements can be made for health organizations to obtain more detailed information. There are confidentiality issues around such statistics and there can be problems with information being out of date by the time it is published; for example, it may be annual data produced several months after a year end, by which time services may have been redesigned.

There are many other examples of government statistics around mental health. Examples include England's mental health minimum dataset (HSCIC n.d. a), which contains record-level data about the care of adults and older people using secondary mental health services. The Welsh Government produces summaries of information on patients admitted to mental health facilities and results of its psychiatric census (Welsh Government n.d.), which covers patients who are resident in NHS mental health hospitals and mental health units in NHS hospitals that may have other specialities. The Scottish Government provides data on its national indicator to improve mental well-being. As with hospital episode statistics, some are only available at high level, and special arrangements may be needed to access more detail.

PRINCIPLES INTO PRACTICE

This chapter has summarized the policy overview, outcomes frameworks and population-based measurement tools currently available for mental health and well-being.

The first of the four principles we set out in the introduction is reflected in this chapter in the way that national policy aspires to promote mental health and well-being holistically. Because certain physical problems such as obesity or long-term conditions can be strongly linked to mental well-being, outcome measures related to these can also be useful indicators. The huge diversity of factors affecting mental health, including the wider determinants reflected in our second principle and discussed further in the next chapter, is also reflected in the range of possible outcome measures. For example, outcome measurements around housing standards, education standards, levels of crime and environmental conditions may all be highly relevant.

While the third principle, that of using health care needs assessment and systematically assessed evidence about what works, is not used directly in this chapter, these two processes underpin the selection and development of outcome frameworks at a national level.

Finally, the fourth principle of community involvement means that outcomes of measures to increase patient or public participation or to reduce discrimination, inequity or inequality can also be very relevant.

Chapter 2

WHAT AFFECTS MENTAL HEALTH AND WELL-BEING?

THE WIDER SOCIAL, CULTURAL AND PHYSICAL ENVIRONMENT

KEY POINTS

- Peace is an essential prerequisite for mental health and well-being.
- The impact of housing on mental health and well-being is increasingly being recognized as vital both as a cause of and a consequence of mental health problems.
- Cross-border flows in goods, services, people and capital affect mental health and well-being in the UK, and ways to maximize benefits of global trade need to be identified.
- There is a complex interaction among inequalities, deprivation, worklessness, education and mental health and well-being.
- Many studies have shown a strong association between access to green and open spaces and to nature, and better mental health.
- Any approach to public mental health should address the challenge of sustainability.
- Those with a mental health problem are more likely to be victims of crime than perpetrators, particularly when it comes to violent crimes.

INTRODUCTION

It has been recognized for a long time that wider economic, environmental and social determinants of health have a major impact on morbidity and mortality (DH 1998). It is not only physical health that is affected: psychosocial reasons are among the commonest reasons for visiting the GP (*ibid.*). Place and space are important for the mental health of individuals and populations (Curtis 2010).

This chapter examines the way in which mental health can be affected by these 'wider determinants' of health. In Chapter 3 we consider the effects of personal circumstances, and in Chapter 4 we consider the impact of individual experience through life stage and lifestyle. The three chapters are closely related. The relationship between wider determinants, personal circumstances and individual experience is fundamental to a population-based understanding of mental health and well-being. This understanding informs practical implications for a wide range of services addressing deprivation, employment, education, housing, crime and the environment. These services may not traditionally see themselves as having a role in creating mental health and well-being, and addressing this challenge is an important one.

We address the issues in an order that broadly mirrors that of the Ottawa Charter prerequisites for health that were outlined in Chapter 1 (peace, shelter, education, food, income, a stable ecosystem, sustainable resources, social justice and equity), although we have subsumed food into a section entitled 'world trade and its impact on mental health'.

PEACE

Peace can be defined as 'a state of quiet; freedom from disturbance, war or contention' (*Chambers Giant Paperback English Dictionary* 1996, p.783).

Proponents of peace see it as a natural state, from which war is a deviation. In Galtung's negative and positive peace framework, negative peace refers to the absence of direct violence and positive peace refers to the absence of indirect and structural violence (Galtung and Jacobsen 2000). One view is that social structures are created through conflict between people with differing interests and resources. Individuals and resources, in turn, are influenced by these structures and by the unequal distribution of power.

An Agenda for Peace is a seminal report written for the United Nations by Secretary-General Boutros Boutros-Ghali in 1992. It contains analysis and recommendations to strengthen peacekeeping in terms of preventive diplomacy, and post-conflict peace-building: 'action to identify and support structures which will tend to strengthen and solidify peace in order to avoid a relapse into conflict' (United Nations General Security Council 1992, p.5).

The Community Foundation for Northern Ireland's *Guide to Peacebuilding in Northern Ireland* states:

> A number of macro issues are currently impacting on peacebuilding practices in Northern Ireland. The sheer magnitude of Peace monies invested in the region, and the fact this funding is currently drawing to a close, has generated increased interest in, and pressure for, collection and sharing of 'best practices' related to peacebuilding. (INCORE & The Community Foundation for Northern Ireland 2006, updated 2010, Interventions Issues, section 7)

One practical aspect of post-conflict peace-building particularly relevant to mental health is supporting victims of torture and violence. One study of the application of brief therapeutic interventions found that:

> despite the fact that the treatment did not notably reduce the symptom experienced by the clients, many had, due to the treatment, found new and better ways of dealing with their pain. Also, since the treatment aimed at strengthening the client's abilities to cope with the complexities of his/her problems on a daily basis, many experienced an increased sense of manageability and meaningfulness in regards to daily life. (Berliner *et al.* 2004)

SHELTER

Good housing and a stable home environment are critical for mental health and well-being. It has long been recognized that inadequate housing can have a major impact on people's physical health: increased incidence of problems such as damp, mould, dust mites and accidents are all related to poor physical health (Wiltshire 2010), and many key public health documents have identified housing as a vital component of good health, from the Black Report (Townsend and Davidson 1982) to the Marmot Review (Marmot 2010b).

In its presentation of the health principles of housing, the WHO states that 'adequate housing helps people's social and psychological development and reduces to a minimum the psychological and social stresses connected with the housing environment' (WHO 1989, p.14). The WHO report suggests that in urban environments, particularly, the housing situation may not be conducive to good mental health. Factors such as overcrowding, noise, crime and uncertainty of tenure are noted as contributing to mental ill health.

A more recent WHO report (2011) describes the way excessive environmental noise (including traffic noise, neighbourhood noise and aircraft noise) acts as a stressor resulting in psychological problems, increased annoyance responses and adverse social behaviour. It mentions also that stressful housing conditions can aggravate pre-existing psychiatric pathologies. Additionally, prolonged heat and cold events can create stress that may exacerbate problems in those with mental health problems or stress-related disorders.

Problems with neighbours can create stress, particularly if someone with a mental health problem faces discrimination from them. This can lead to people feeling unsafe in their homes (Mind n.d. b).

The impact of housing on mental health and well-being has increasingly been recognized as vital both as a cause of and a consequence of mental health problems. Poor-quality housing (for example, dwellings that are damp, lack security or have high levels of noise) is particularly associated with depression (BMA 2003; Hopton and Hunt 1996). The decrease in social housing and the affordability crisis are leading to overcrowding, with its detrimental effect on family relationships and the emotional development of children (Dockery et al. 2010).

People with mental health problems are particularly at risk with regard to housing, often because they are unable to secure and maintain appropriate accommodation. Mental illness can lead to a range of problems that might culminate in job loss; inability to maintain rent or mortgage payments then leads to the loss of home and possible relationship breakdown (Appleton and Molyneux 2011). Homelessness is discussed further in Chapter 3. Mental ill health is often given as a reason for tenancy breakdown (Social Exclusion Unit 2004). Poor mental health, lack of work, inadequate housing and income poverty combine to leave people experiencing 'multiple disadvantage' – 'Multiple disadvantage refers to individuals or families who experience two or more disadvantages, such as low income, poor health and no qualifications' (Cabinet Office 2010, p.59). People with mental health problems are one and a half times more likely than the general population to live in rented housing, twice as likely to be unhappy with their accommodation and four times more likely to consider that their housing makes their health worse (Johnson, Griffiths and Nottingham 2006). Problems with housing are often cited as a reason for admission into inpatient mental health care (*ibid.*).

The welfare reforms of 2013 are likely to exacerbate housing problems. The government amalgamated benefits to provide one monthly payment for claimants. This includes rent, which was previously paid directly to the landlord. Benefit recipients are expected to budget 'responsibly'. The government tested out the new system and it was shown that tenants had limited or no experience of managing a monthly budget, did not have bank accounts, and it was clear that when money was very limited rent may have lower priority than providing food for the children (BBC 2012).

EDUCATION

Education is critical to individual and societal well-being. As the New Economics Foundation states:

> Learning encourages social interaction and increases self-esteem and feelings of competency. Behaviour directed by personal goals to achieve something new has been shown to increase reported life satisfaction. While there is often a much greater policy emphasis on learning in the early years of life, psychological research suggests it is a critical aspect of day-to-day living for all age groups. (Michaelson *et al.* 2009, p.46)

Poor mental health has been consistently linked with poor educational attainment and high rates of drop out from education (Cornaglia, Crivellaro and McNally 2012). The crucial role of social, behavioural and cognitive development on positive educational outcomes at the start of school has been demonstrated, particularly in relation to independence and concentration (Friedli 2009).

Within school, conduct problems, which are common, cover a range of antisocial forms of behaviour, including disobedience, lying, fighting and stealing. Colman *et al.* (2009) found that 6 per cent of children aged 5–10 years had a severe conduct problem and 19 per cent had mild conduct problems. By adolescence, the rates had risen to 9 per cent and 29 per cent respectively, and those with severe problems were more likely to leave school without any qualifications (65%) compared to those with mild problems (52%) and those with none (31%).

Other problems that young people suffer include anxiety and depression, which can have a significant impact on exam performance. This is associated with loss of confidence or self-esteem, excessive worrying, lack of pleasure and a lack of interest in usual activities (Cornaglia *et al.* 2012). Low educational attainment is linked to lower rates of engagement in education of any kind or in employment and to a risk of subsequent poor mental health. However, even average levels of educational achievement do not guarantee average rates of people in education or employment. In the UK, 11 per cent of 11–18 year-olds are not in education, employment or training (NEET), a much higher rate than in several other countries, despite reaching similar levels of educational standards (ONS 2012b).

WORLD TRADE AND ITS IMPACT ON MENTAL HEALTH

Seeking improved health and increased income have long been common goals. Those who make the case that free trade will help everyone argue that the growth from increased trade will be shared and will improve people's lives. But they have not answered the fundamental question of how to formulate trade policy simultaneously to achieve growth and benefit health. *Trade and Health* explores all the avenues through which trade affects health, and examines a number of case studies on how best to achieve policies that integrate health objectives (Blouin, Heymann and Drager 2007).

Cross-border flows in goods, services, people and capital are affecting health through an increasing number of channels. Examples of each of these that are related to mental health in the UK include: flow of illicit drugs, cheap food, alcohol and tobacco into the country; flow of health professionals into and out of the country; and flow of trafficked people, asylum-seekers and refugees into the country. UK financial services are key to the global economy. Trade agreements have implications for health and the health sector, whether they are multilateral, bilateral or linked to the World Trade Organization (WTO) or regional trading systems (WHO 2009a).

The World Health Organization is developing a diagnostic tool and companion workbook that will guide national policymakers building public policies and strategies related to trade and health (*ibid.*).

INCOME (EMPLOYMENT AND UNEMPLOYMENT)

Bambra (2011) describes work as being of value in three ways: economically, as self-identity and as part of a social contract. She states that worklessness as a term is most often used in the UK to refer to people out of work and in receipt of welfare benefits for one of three reasons: unemployment, lone parenthood or ill health. While on the one hand almost everyone of working age is expected to work, or at least be economically active, full employment is no longer considered a feasible goal. Structural worklessness is therefore an issue, which states address in different ways, involving the social security system, the labour market and the organization of work. Policy interventions may mediate the relationships between work, worklessness and health inequalities. For example, 'the relationship between job insecurity and poor health is less in those countries with more extensive social systems which improve the ability of individuals to cope with stressful events' (p.190). Health-related worklessness is more than 50 per cent among people with a chronic illness in countries where state provision is minimal and benefits have strict entitlement criteria; it is less than 40 per cent in welfare states where social rights are available to all socio-economic groups. The socio-economic consequences of ill health are also higher in the first group of countries than in the second. This is discussed further in Chapter 6 under 'Build healthy public policy'.

Work, worklessness and health are strongly interrelated: unemployment has been recognized as having major links with poor mental health, and the importance of work in maintaining good mental health has been highlighted (e.g. Gillborn 2008). Paul and Moser (2009) found that 34 per cent of unemployed people had psychological problems, compared with 16 per cent of those in work. Those with mental illness who are unemployed are less likely to recover (Singleton and Lewis 2003). Not only is poor mental health associated with unemployment, but unemployment itself can lead to increased poor outcomes, such as substance abuse, crime and suicidal thoughts (Fergusson, Horwood and Woodward 2001).

The beneficial effects of work outweigh the risks and are greater than the harmful effects of long-term unemployment and prolonged sickness absence (Black and Frost 2011). Waddell and Burton's (2006) review found that for most people:

- work is beneficial to well-being and health
- unemployment is detrimental to well-being and health
- re-employment leads to improved health; further unemployment leads to deterioration
- work improves the health and psychosocial status of sick or disabled individuals
- moving off benefit improves health, including the health of those with severe mental health problems
- there is no evidence that work is harmful to the mental health of people with severe mental illness.

The 2007 Adult Psychiatric Morbidity Survey (NHSIC 2009) found that, in England, poverty and unemployment tended to increase the duration of episodes of common mental disorders. Unemployment was also found to be linked to less common mental health disorders. This is a complex issue, because people may be less likely to be in paid employment as a consequence of pre-existing mental illness. Alternatively, unemployment may lead to deterioration in mental health.

For most people, employment is beneficial. Unfortunately, there are some for whom work can be a negative stressor, with stress, depression and anxiety together being the greatest cause of sickness absence (Friedli 2009). Lower job satisfaction can lead to lower productivity and also reduced well-being, which may be caused by workplaces that 'sap morale and energy' (Black 2008, p.32). Changes to the physical and psychosocial work environments, such as increasing workers' control and participation, have been shown to improve occupational health (Bambra 2011).

Many people with mental health problems are particularly disadvantaged when it comes to employment (Butterworth *et al.* 2012; Social Exclusion Unit 2004): although many want to work, they have the lowest employment rate for any of the main disability groups, with less than one-quarter working. Once unemployed, individuals with poor mental health are less likely to get paid work than those without such problems (Butterworth *et al.* 2012). Only 4 in 10 employers are prepared to engage someone with such problems, compared to 6 in 10 who are prepared to employ someone with physical health problems (Social Exclusion Unit 2004). In this context, people might be reluctant to disclose their psychiatric history when applying for jobs.

If individuals with mental health problems obtain employment, they are more likely to be underemployed or employed in low-status and low-paid jobs (Stuart 2006) and less likely to be offered training or promotion (Michalak *et al.* 2007). They are likely to be more closely questioned on return from sickness for a mental illness, as well as to be demoted or even dismissed (Baldwin and Marcus 2006): a third of employers have been found not to believe information on a sick note from an employee with a mental health problem (Manning and White 1995). A person with mental health problems is more than twice as likely to leave employment as someone with other health conditions (Burchardt 2003).

Unemployment through poor mental health can have a huge impact on the financial situation of an individual and family. It can lead to income loss, debt, poverty and deprivation, with impacts on mental health as discussed in the previous section. Additionally, most people achieve through work a level of financial status to allow full participation in society. Those without work who have mental health problems are therefore doubly stigmatized (McCrone *et al.* 2008): both unemployment and social isolation are major risk factors for deteriorating mental health.

A STABLE ECOSYSTEM AND SUSTAINABLE RESOURCES

The wider environment and climate change

The biophysical environment, including climate change and other aspects of environmental degradation, is now recognized as a determinant of health. Even if addressed as a matter of urgency, the deteriorating state of Earth's surface and biosphere will discriminate against future generations (Graham 2012). Earth's rising surface temperature and the resultant melting of the world's ice sheets are causing sea levels to rise, making huge areas at risk of floods, droughts and other severe weather events (Committee on America's Climate Choices 2011; Pachauri and Reisinger 2007).

The severe weather changes are likely to affect farming and fishing detrimentally, with falling crop yields potentially leading to food scarcity, which is more likely to affect the most deprived communities (Ebmeier 2012). Frequent flooding and warmer weather are likely to lead to an increased number of physical health issues (*ibid.*). From a mental health perspective, extreme weather will have an impact on people's coping mechanisms, with the outcomes being long-term stress, anxiety and depression (Pitt 2008).

No one organization or sector can solve all the problems of climate change. At a local level, emergency plans can take into account the increased frequency of extreme weather conditions (North East Climate Change Partnership 2008), but some aspects need a global approach (Committee on America's Climate Choices 2011). Acheson (1988, p.1) defined public health as 'the science and art of preventing disease, prolonging life, and promoting health through organized efforts of society'. Graham (2012) proposes that tackling the issue of the deteriorating state of Earth's surface and biosphere should be central to public health activity as part of the organized efforts of society, involving people and organizations at all levels.

Sustainability

Hanlon *et al.* (2013) argue that there is a need for a new approach to public health that is capable of addressing the challenge of sustainability, through offering a new world view to take the place of 'modernism'. This approach applies the following five criteria. It would be:

- integrative, making moral decisions based on both science and aesthetics
- ecological, using a systems approach to mimic natural complex adaptive systems
- ethical, in terms of our individual rights and collective imperatives
- creative, because we need to imagine something better
- beautiful, in order to raise our spirits.

Graham (2012) also argues that public health stewardship should centrally include issues of sustainability; its duty is to protect conditions for health over time and across generations. She argues that current research methods are ill suited to thinking about future risks. The 'discounting' of future benefits traditional in health economics is based on research asking people if they would like jam (or its equivalent) now or next week. There have been very few studies asking people how much they care about future generations.

Today's population is the privileged minority; the disadvantaged majority has yet to be born. Future generations have moral equality with those currently alive (HM Treasury 2006; later published as Stern 2007). We borrow environmental capital from future generations with no intention or ability to repay it. An intergenerational perspective on inequality, putting future generations' moral claims on to the agenda, would help us to recognize the biophysical environment as a determinant of health, and so focus our attention on the stability of Earth's surface environment.

Local environment

Where people live is intimately related to their housing and socio-economic circumstances, which then relates to the work that they are able to participate in, if, indeed, there is any work available (Barnard and Turner 2011). Other important factors include lack of amenities, poor social resources, and an area of high crime, or one that is perceived as being so (Batty et al. 2010).

There is generally growing evidence of the importance of the physical environment for mental health, although establishing a causal link is difficult (Curtis 2010; Flach et al. 2011; Mass et al. 2006). In this subsection, we consider the very local environment, following on from the wider environmental issue of global climate change looked at above.

A recent study (Nettle et al. 2014) found that the residents of a deprived neighbourhood had lower levels of social trust and higher levels of paranoia than the residents of an affluent neighbourhood. Furthermore, visitors to the two neighbourhoods who were only there for 45 minutes mirrored the differences seen in the residents.

Cognitive, affective and behavioural benefits have been recognized. Impacts include: 'fostering psychological well-being; increased life satisfaction, self-esteem and self-confidence; increased positive mood states and decreased negative emotions such as anger; reduced anxiety; reduced stress and an aid to coping as an escape from daily stresses' (Parkinson 2007, p.50).

There is some evidence of mental health benefits to children of regular access to natural environments: reduced symptoms among children with attention deficit hyperactivity disorder; increased concentration and self-discipline among inner-city girls; enhanced emotional and values-related development in schoolchildren; and reduced stress in children in rural areas (FPH 2013).

Many studies have shown a strong association between access to green and open spaces and to nature, and better mental health (Clarke *et al.* 2007). Green space can provide a buffer against the negative health effects of stressful events (van den Berg *et al.* 2010). In an exploration of the benefits of green space to mental health, Grahn and Stigsdotter (2010) found that serenity was the most important element in providing a restorative environment for individuals who were stressed. Viewing greenery, rather than concrete, increases concentration and reduces aggression. Experimental studies on volunteers have shown a reduction in measured physiological stress indicators (e.g. electroencephalogram (EEG) alpha-wave activity, skin conductance, blood pressure) during nature viewing compared to a rise during non-nature viewing (FPH 2013).

Crime and domestic violence in families with views of vegetation are reduced by 50 per cent (Kuo and Sullivan 2001). People travelling to work on nature-dominated routes had much lower stress rates than those travelling through built-up areas. It also reduces hospital stays and the need for pain relief (Bird 2007). Barton and Pretty (2010) found that all green environments had a positive effect on both mood and self-esteem. The presence of water had even greater effects. Perceived greenness has been found to be associated more strongly with mental health than physical health (Sugiyama *et al.* 2008).

Mental illness is more prevalent in urban areas (Morrissey *et al.* 2012), and mental health is better in rural areas, with the strongest evidence being for psychosis, particularly schizophrenia (Nicholson 2008; SAMH 2012). The situation, however, is complicated, as it appears that some with chronic mental health problems may move into urban areas to get better access to mental health services (Nicholson 2008).

The exception to better mental health is around suicide, where rural rates are higher, in part because 'farming communities, and farmers and vets in particular, have ready access to firearms and drugs if seeking to take their own lives' (Wood 2004).

The positive impact that any physical activity has on mental well-being has been well documented (APHO 2007; Biddle 2000; Halliwell 2005) and is further discussed in Chapter 5. So in terms of mental health, the advantages of green spaces appear twofold: green spaces improve mental health and have the added advantage of increasing physical activity, which in turn has a strong impact on mental health and well-being.

SOCIAL JUSTICE AND EQUITY

Deprivation and poverty

The relationship between high levels of deprivation and high rates of mental ill health is well established, with an increased risk of mental ill health for the poor when compared with the non-poor (Payne 2000). As Weich and Lewis (1998) comment, 'financial strain is a powerful independent predictor of both the onset and maintenance of episodes of common mental disorders, even after adjusting for more objective measures of standard of living' (p.118).

Because poor people often live in poor areas, combinations of material and social deprivation may emerge. For example, in neighbourhoods with a lack of material resources, physical deterioration of the built environment may engender unease or even fear, and can create a stigma around the area. Individual mental health is affected by social circumstances along a spectrum from social support/cohesion to isolation/fragmentation, alongside material living conditions along a spectrum from comfortable/secure/safe to insecure/uncomfortable (Curtis 2010).

Certain items in a list of basic necessities have been found to be more associated with poor mental health than others. Payne (2000) found that more than 70 per cent of people with poor mental health had no access to fresh fruit and vegetables, while more than 65 per cent did not have a warm waterproof coat. In itself, this can contribute to poorer physical health, but there is also evidence that chronic stress, such as that linked with living in poverty, has adverse effects on physical health.

The association between problematic social aspects of life, living in poverty, consequent stress and poor physical health has been mapped in terms of the body's physiological response to prolonged stress. Chronic stress has an impact on the cardiovascular, the neuro-endocrine and the immune systems, by affecting hormone levels, which influence blood pressure, cholesterol levels and inflammation (Friedli 2009). Physical ill health, as well as poverty, can increase mental ill health and stress, with stress having an impact on memory and on the risk of depression and post-traumatic stress syndrome (Wolf and Buss 2009).

While poverty overall is very strongly linked to mental health problems, there are particular issues also surrounding debt and its management (with potential approaches to this discussed in Chapter 6). A 2012 survey found that three-quarters of respondents said that debt worries were affecting their health, with problems including panic or anxiety attacks (Citizens Advice 2012).

The interrelationship between mental health and debt is well recognized:

> Sadly financial problems and mental health are a marriage made in hell. Each ride off the back of the other. The net result is that a hugely disproportionate number of people with mental health problems face severe debt crisis. Not just because poor money management, impulse and emotional control are often symptoms of mental health problems – but because these health issues hit income too. (Lewis 2013, p.3)

For those with debt problems, payday loans can create serious problems. These loans, currently under investigation by the Competition Commission, are designed for short-term borrowing and have very high interest. Access to them is said to be easy, apparently without appropriate financial checks, so that very desperate people, including those with mental health problems, can obtain loans (e.g. BBC 2013a) and find that their debt problems can worsen significantly. This exacerbates the stress and is likely to make mental health problems worse.

Another potential financial difficulty for those with mental health problems arises in trying to get insurance (e.g. Mind n.d. a). Insurance companies assess the risk of customers using a series of questions, but it is believed that there are some companies that do not ask the right questions about the risks of many mental health problems.

Answering 'yes' to a single question asking whether the applicant has ever had a mental health problem can lead to a refusal to provide cover. Non-disclosure is not an option as it can invalidate any policy. There are some relevant laws that help to protect against discrimination, but there are also exemptions. Trying to obtain insurance can exacerbate stress-related problems, and being without insurance can also be very worrying, especially if problems arise and property or possessions are lost.

Socio-economic status

People living in households with the lowest levels of income in England are more likely to have a common mental disorder (anxiety or depression) than those living in the highest income households (NHSIC 2009). The prevalence of psychotic disorder has also been found to vary by level of income, increasing from 0.1 per cent of adults in the highest income quintile to 0.9 per cent of adults in the lowest income quintile. This trend was more prominent among men than women. There are higher rates of psychiatric admissions and suicides in areas of high deprivation and unemployment (Boardman *et al.* 1997; Croudace *et al.* 2000; Gunnell *et al.* 1995; Kammerling and O'Connor 1993). People living in 'economic hardship' on a long-term basis are more likely to be suffering from clinical depression, anxiety and phobias (Lynch, Kaplan and Shema 1997; Meltzer, Gill and Petticrew 1995).

The links between poor health and deprivation have been shown to be strong, but it is *relative* poverty that causes many problems in Western societies, rather than absolute poverty (Wilkinson 2005; Wilkinson and Pickett 2009), and 'the prevalence of mental illness is much more acute in countries with high income inequality' (Wilkinson 2007, p.6).

Wilkinson (2005) argues that inequalities in income encourage suspicion, distrust and hostility and therefore limit social integration and participation. Within Western societies, income is a marker for social status. Individuals acquire status through being rich. It is not just worries about having enough money, but the feelings of being looked down on, of being devalued and treated as a second-class citizen, that is so detrimental to health. Mental well-being has been found to be positively associated with the perceived quality of the home at a local level, the desirability of the home, the reputation of the neighbourhood and the standard of living (Kearns *et al.* 2013).

More equal societies, where income differentials are smallest between the rich and poor, have greater social cohesion and trust. There are lower levels of hostility, violence and homicide and, in turn, this is linked with lower rates of poor mental health and decreased susceptibility to heart disease (Cooper *et al.* 1999). There is a strong correlation between reported levels of social trust and measures of well-being (Kawachi, Kennedy and Lochner 1997) and strong evidence that living within a society that has fewer inequalities has a positive impact on mental health: the chronic stress caused by struggling with material disadvantage is exacerbated by living in an unequal society (Friedli 2009). Groups with the lowest incomes in the most unequal societies are thus likely to be the most at risk of consequent health problems (Wilkinson 2005).

From a preventive perspective, the Marmot Review (Marmot 2010b) focused on how health inequalities are not inevitable and how action can, and should, be taken to address them, for strong social, as well as economic, reasons. This is discussed further in Chapter 5 under 'Build healthy public policy'. Marmot found that innate cognitive ability at birth can be reduced or increased dramatically by the age of two, depending on the social environment. This affects the child's life chances in ways that are discussed in Chapter 3, and has implications for service delivery, as discussed in Chapter 6.

Crime

There are several myths around the prevalence of violent crime and mental illness, as well as a range of related issues about stigma and discrimination.

The Poverty and Social Exclusion Survey (Payne 2000) found that those who were poor were more likely than wealthier respondents to have been burgled, to have had their houses or cars deliberately damaged, and to have experienced personal theft. Not only was the experience of crime greater within deprived communities, but fear of crime was greatest in this group, particularly among the poor and elderly (*ibid.*): 37 per cent of those living in poverty reported feeling unsafe walking out in the dark, compared with 27 per cent of the non-poor. Payne also found that twice as many of those who were poor and felt unsafe going out in the dark also had mental health problems, when compared with the more affluent. This may be partly because people with less income have less access to a car or the resources to pay for a taxi. Added to this, areas of high deprivation tend to have higher crime rates (Mooney and Neal 2010). So those living in poverty are more likely than the average to be victims of crime, and areas of high deprivation are also more likely to have high rates of poor mental health. Consequently, areas with high levels of crime are likely to have higher levels of mental illness (APHO 2007).

There is a widespread belief that people with mental illness are prone to violence and more likely to commit violent crime (Mental Health Reporting 2013). However, the majority of people who commit violent crime do not suffer from mental illness, and the risk of violence from people who are mentally ill is very small (*ibid.*). The contribution of people with mental health problems to overall rates of violence is small, and the extent of the relationship is greatly exaggerated in the minds of the general public. Much of the information that the public get about mental illness is from the media. Wahl, Wood and Richards (2002) found that newspapers carried twice as many negative articles about violence and mental health problems as positive ones, thus perpetuating fears within communities.

Indeed, it is worth noting that those with a mental health problem are more likely to be victims of crime than perpetrators, particularly when it comes to violent crimes (Appleby *et al.* 2001). Hiday (2006) found that people with severe mental illnesses, such as schizophrenia, bipolar disorder or other psychosis, are themselves two and a half times more likely to be attacked, mugged or raped than the rest of the population. There are, however, links between non-violent crime and poor mental health, with offenders being more likely to suffer mental health problems. (The mental health of offenders is discussed in Chapter 3.)

PRINCIPLES INTO PRACTICE

This chapter has focused particularly on our second principle: it is vital to address the social, economic, political, cultural and environmental factors that enhance mental health and well-being, the 'determinants of health'. The next two chapters will pick up the thread in terms of the first principle: mental health and well-being is central to an individual's social purpose, autonomy and ability to make life choices, and, in turn, is affected by them. There is a complex two-way interaction between the wider determinants of health with their impact on individuals, and vice versa.

Chapter 3

WHAT AFFECTS MENTAL HEALTH AND WELL-BEING?

INDIVIDUAL SOCIAL, CULTURAL AND PHYSICAL CIRCUMSTANCES

KEY POINTS

Life circumstances can have a profound effect:

- Events such as bereavement, sexual abuse or exploitation, domestic violence and becoming a refugee or homeless all increase the risk of mental illness, particularly depression.

- Discrimination and abuse can cause mental health problems in groups with different sexuality or ethnicity.

- Divorced people, carers and children in a family unit with stepbrothers and stepsisters have higher risks of poor mental health.

- People who have been in the armed forces, in prison or in the 'looked-after' system are particularly vulnerable to mental health problems.

- People with long-term conditions and physical or learning disability are at risk of mental health problems such as depression.

- Mental health is adversely affected by many factors, but it also influences many of them. Social isolation contributes to depression, but those with depression are less likely to be socially active.

INTRODUCTION

Chapter 2 described the way in which mental health can be affected by external factors, such as the economy or the environment. In this chapter and the following one, we consider factors that are more specific to individuals in terms of the effects they have on mental well-being and the scale of the mental health problem. Successful approaches or guidance to improving the situation are discussed in Chapter 6. Some of the factors are discussed in more detail in the later extended case-study chapters (Chapters 7, 8 and 9), but here, because of the huge range of issues, descriptions are necessarily brief and are intended merely to give a flavour of the influential factors.

The topics in this chapter are arranged alphabetically, and the varying lengths of the sections do not signify that some are more important than others but generally reflect the extent of available relevant material. Where issues are more pertinent to one of our case studies (suicide, people with long-term conditions and young Black and Minority Ethnic (BME) groups), they are discussed there.

BEREAVEMENT

Bereavement is a complex and highly individual experience, and is different for everyone. Grief, a person's experience of loss, can include physical symptoms, such as changes in appetite and weight, fatigue and sleep loss, nausea and headache. It also includes emotional and spiritual reactions, such as sadness and pain, and can be exacerbated by the experience of nursing people through a final illness (NICE 2004a).

The extent to which bereavement is considered a mental health problem in itself has been debated. It is generally accepted that there is a grief pattern that is 'normal' within certain parameters. Kleinman (2012) identified the lack of a 'normal' time period, but noted that the fourth version of the *Diagnostic and Statistical Manual of Mental Disorders* (DSM-IV) classified depressive-type symptoms as a result of bereavement lasting beyond two months to be appropriate for a diagnosis of depression. With DSM-5 this exclusion of the first two months was removed, to try to help prevent major depression being overlooked (American Psychiatric Association 2013b). Shear *et al.* (2011) suggest that, although most people are resilient to the experience of bereavement, people with an increased risk of mental illness or those experiencing poor mental health can be negatively affected, and some 10 per cent of bereaved people are affected by chronic grief. These people would benefit from treatment (Kleinman 2012).

Bereavement can lead to loneliness and isolation, particularly in older people already suffering from the effects of ill health and poverty. This is exacerbated by the changing family structure of current times, with people living longer and having smaller families, who often live at a distance from their parents (Griffin 2010).

Children and young people will experience some sort of depression as they grieve, even if they do not fully understand the reality of death; even babies can feel loss (Cruse n.d.). It is natural for them to feel confused and there can be anxiety that someone else may die or that they may forget what the deceased person looked like; this anxiety can lead to episodes of depression (*ibid.*).

Where someone is bereaved by the death of someone serving in the armed forces, they may have particular issues and experiences that can complicate the grieving process. Because serving personnel tend to be young, there are often children affected by the bereavement (*ibid.*). Other traumatic losses include death from natural disaster, violence or suicide (*ibid.*). Each of these may give rise to specific problems, and the bereaved may need help or advice from sources focused on the manner of death.

BLACK AND MINORITY ETHNIC GROUPS

Issues around mental health for BME groups are discussed in our case study in Chapter 8.

BULLYING

Oxford Dictionaries (n.d.) defines a bully as 'a person who uses strength of influence to harm or intimidate those who are weaker'. Examples of bullying include treating someone unfairly, spreading unpleasant rumours, undermining or picking on someone, and denying opportunities to a person (Gov.UK 2014).

Adi *et al.* (2007) found that approximately half of primary school children were bullied regularly and that children who are violent and aggressive and who bully have been shown to come from backgrounds where aggression is used as the favoured problem-solving method. Bullying has widespread effects on the health of victims, including depressive and anxiety symptoms and suicidal thoughts (*ibid.*).

Almost 16,000 pupils are absent from school as a consequence of bullying at any one time (Brown, Clery and Ferguson 2011). There is growing evidence that bullying is linked to mental health problems. One study found that 61.5 per cent of adolescents attending mental health services for children and young people reported that bullying was an important reason for their attendance at those services (Dyer and Teggart 2007).

Adults also experience bullying. Most research has focused on the workplace and shows that, although 85 per cent of organizations have anti-bullying policies, it is still a huge issue, costing employers upwards of £2 billion per year (Tehrani 2005).

Cyber-bullying is a problem on the increase and affects everyone, although young people are particularly at risk. Cyber-bullying (online bullying) is when a person or a group of people use the Internet, email, online games or any other kind of digital technology to threaten, tease, upset or humiliate someone else.

Many groups are at particular risk of bullying, including:

- disabled people (Hoong Sin *et al.* 2009)
- people with learning disabilities (Mencap 2007; Quarmby 2011)
- LGBT people (Aspinall and Mitton 2008)
- BME people (RCPsych 2010).

CARERS

Carers look after an ill, disabled or frail family member, friend or partner without pay (Carers UK 2012). In England, there are about five million carers (12 per cent of people older than 16 years) (NHSIC 2010), and with increasingly large numbers of older people in the population, this number is expected to rise considerably over the coming years. More than a third of carers provide care for more than 20 hours per week, and almost a quarter provide more than 50 hours' care per week (Carers UK 2012).

Women are more likely to be carers than men, with approximately 60 per cent of carers being female (NHSIC 2010). The number of carers more than 65 years of age is increasing at the greatest rate, and middle-aged people are most likely to be caring for dependent children as well as older adults (Agree, Bissett and Rendall 2003). The number of young carers, under 18 years, was estimated at 175,000 in the 2001 Census, although broader definitions indicate much higher numbers (Carers UK 2012). In terms of ethnicity, Bangladeshi and Pakistani people are three times more likely to be carers than the white population (Yeandle, Stiell and Buckner 2006).

The mental health of carers can be seriously affected by their being on a lower income, because of the reduced opportunities to work. Disability benefits often will not cover the additional household and living expenses resulting from poor health and disability, such as travel, heating and laundry costs. Carers UK (2011) found that nearly two-thirds of carers use their own money to provide such essentials.

The responsibility of caring can affect both physical and mental health. Those caring for more than 50 hours a week are twice as likely to be in poor physical health as non-carers, particularly problematic in younger carers (Carers UK 2004). This situation is mirrored as far as poor mental health is concerned, with carers being more than twice as likely as non-carers to experience poor mental health (Singleton *et al.* 2002). This includes high levels of depression, anxiety and loss of confidence and self-esteem (Carers UK 2004).

Carers experience high levels of isolation, with more than half blaming lack of support from health or social care services (Contact a Family 2011). Carers UK (2012) found that 4 in 10 had not had a full day off from caring within the last year and half had not had a holiday away from home for at least five years. Moreover, 66 per cent of carers reported that caring had a negative impact on friendships, and a further 58 per cent reported that caring adversely affected their relationships with other family members. The importance of social relationships to good mental and emotional health is further discussed in the section on social isolation and inclusion.

FAMILY SIZE AND STRUCTURE

Families with a larger number of children are more likely to experience domestic violence, which has an impact on children's mental health

(Meltzer *et al.* 2009). However, family size correlates with a range of other factors that impact on mental health, particularly poverty.

Lone parents are more likely than any other group to suffer from depression. This is related to poverty and social exclusion (Brown and Moran 1997), but these factors do not explain the full extent of depression found in this group (Hope, Power and Rodgers 1999).

Adults living in family units with children have a higher risk of depression than those without children, although it has been suggested that this may relate to high levels of lone parenthood (Payne 2000). In couples with children, both partners have higher rates of depression than couples without children (Meltzer *et al.* 1995).

Women across all marital status categories are more likely than their male counterparts to have a common mental health condition (mainly anxiety or depression), except for divorced people, in whom the prevalence for men and women was very similar (27%) (NHSIC 2009). The highest rates of psychotic disorder have been found among those who are divorced, and the lowest rates among those who are married (*ibid.*).

The prevalence of eating disorder has been found to vary by marital status, being most common among single men and women (particularly women) and least common among the widowed group, although the variation is likely to be due at least in part to the age profile of the different marital status groups (*ibid.*).

Divorced adults are most likely to have thought about suicide at some point in their life (three times as likely in the case of men), and suicide attempts are also more common in divorced adults than among other adults (*ibid.*). Again, this may be related to the age profile of the different marital status groups.

HOMELESSNESS

Homelessness can be both a cause and a consequence of major problems for an individual's health, both physical and mental. It can make it very difficult for people to get employment or to access services. People with mental health problems may find it difficult to deal with daily living and paying rent, leading to homelessness, which in turn can contribute to mental ill health (Crisis 2011).

A third to a half of homeless people sleeping rough have mental health problems. Common mental health problems are twice as likely and psychosis up to 15 times more likely than in the general population. Homelessness is a hugely stressful situation and can lead to depression and anxiety, with mothers and children suffering significantly higher levels of mental health problems (Suglia, Duarte and Sandel 2011).

Homeless young people are particularly vulnerable: the experience of homelessness can exacerbate existing mental health problems or contribute to the onset of mental health problems, and mental health problems are also a risk factor for homelessness (Mental Health Foundation 2002). In common with many young people, they may have difficulty expressing their needs but, unlike most young people, they may have no responsible adults to advocate on their behalf (*ibid.*). Unaccompanied asylum-seekers and refugees may be even more vulnerable than other young people (*ibid.*).

Drug misuse is common (70%) in homeless rough sleepers (Mental Health Foundation 2007). Four out of five people start using at least one new drug after becoming homeless, sometimes as a coping mechanism, and drug and alcohol abuse account for more than a third of all deaths in the homeless (Crisis 2011). It is more difficult for homeless people to access services to help them to manage their drug and alcohol problems (*ibid.*).

Suicide rates are high, with homeless people more than nine times more likely to commit suicide than the general population (*ibid.*).

It is known that homelessness in women tends to be under-recorded because they are less likely to sleep rough for safety reasons, and more likely to be a part of the 'hidden-homeless' population – staying with others, often in exchange for sex (WHEC 2013).

LOOKED-AFTER CHILDREN

In the UK in 2012 there were more than 91,000 looked-after children, more than half of whom became looked after because of abuse or neglect (NSPCC 2011). More than 70 per cent are cared for by foster carers; more than 10 per cent live in residential homes (almost all more than the age of ten); 8 per cent live with parents subject to a care order; and a small number live in secure children's homes (Mooney *et al.* 2009). Nearly a third are placed outside of their local authority boundary (*ibid.*).

It is wrong to assume that all children in care are kept safe. A minority are at continued risk of abuse or neglect, including from their carers, other young people and those in the wider community who target them. (NSPCC 2011)

Estimates have suggested that half of looked-after children have a mental health disorder (five times the proportion in children generally), and the situation is even worse (more than 70%) for those in residential care (Mooney *et al.* 2009). Even before becoming looked-after children, most will have experienced many more problems than other children – for instance, neglect, abuse or bereavement. The change to their living circumstances, perhaps leaving a family home, can be very unsettling (Mental Health Foundation 2002).

One major study found that the most common diagnosis in looked-after adolescents was conduct disorders, followed by over-anxious disorder. Almost a quarter suffered from major depressive disorders (compared with only 4 per cent of children generally), and 8 per cent had been diagnosed with psychosis (*ibid.*). Possibly already suffering the stigma of being looked after, children can feel more stigmatized if they are also diagnosed with a mental health problem (*ibid.*).

Looked-after children have higher than average children's rates of smoking, illicit drug usage and obesity (Mooney *et al.* 2009), all of which are linked with higher rates of mental health problems (as will be discussed in the 'Personal behaviours' section of Chapter 4). Educational achievement is considerably lower in looked-after children; for example, in 2010 only 26 per cent of looked-after children gained five or more A–C grades at Key Stage 4, compared to 75 per cent of all pupils (DfE 2011). As was mentioned in the previous chapter, poor educational attainment is very much linked to poor mental health and is more likely to lead to difficulties in getting employment and a greater likelihood of poverty, which again has strong associations with poor mental health.

Problems continue when children leave care, with higher rates of earlier parenthood, more drug and alcohol problems and a greater prevalence of both physical and mental health problems (Mooney *et al.* 2009).

Looked-after children may not have anyone to confide in, particularly if they are constantly being moved between placements or if there is not consistency in staff or social workers. This may mean that they are short of adult help in getting support for any mental illness (Mental Health Foundation 2002). In 2009/2010, 1 in 26 of all looked-after children in the UK was counselled by ChildLine (NSPCC 2011). Multiple placements may also mean that even if a child has begun this with Child and Adolescent Mental Health Services, contact is lost because the child is moved to a different area.

OFFENDERS

In May 2012 there were approximately 94,000 prisoners in England, Wales and Scotland (Prison Reform Trust 2012). The prevalence of mental health problems (particularly psychosis, personality disorder and depression or anxiety) in prisons (prisoners aged 16 years and over) is far higher than the prevalence in the general population (aged 16–64 years) (Centre for Mental Health updated 2011). The vast majority of prisoners (over 90%) have a range of psychiatric disorders, including drug and alcohol dependence, neurotic conditions, psychotic illness and personality disorders, and those on remand have higher rates than sentenced prisoners (Bradley 2009).

Not only do high numbers of people with a mental health problem enter prison, some develop depression or anxiety while in prison (Joint Committee on Human Rights 2004). There are high levels of self-harm and suicide within prisons. In the community, self-harm is common but often covert. In prisons, such incidents are more likely to be detected and counted (MoJ 2011). In 2010, the Ministry of Justice reported 58 prison suicides and nearly 27,000 episodes of self-harm (Centre for Mental Health updated 2011).

Prisoners are often disadvantaged by their social circumstances before coming into contact with the criminal justice system. Many are unemployed before going to prison (Social Exclusion Unit 2002); truancy, lack of qualifications and lack of basic numeracy and literacy are common, and up to half have no fixed abode (Centre for Mental Health updated 2011). Once people have a criminal record, they continue to be disadvantaged. In particular, offenders are often excluded from employment and training opportunities. Although being in work reduces re-offending in a range from 30 per cent to 50 per cent (Social Exclusion Unit 2002), only a few prisoners have jobs to go to on release (NCCMH 2010a).

Some groups are particularly at risk of mental health problems within the criminal justice system, including women, people from

BME communities, young people and people with learning disabilities (Commission for Healthcare Audit and Inspection 2007; MoJ 2010; Prison Reform Trust 2011). Although women make up less than 5 per cent of prisoners, they account for almost half of all reported self-harm episodes: 37 per cent self-harmed, compared to 7 per cent of male prisoners. In comparison, the 95 per cent of suicides in custody were male in 2009 (MoJ 2011). This is a greater gender division than that in the general population, where the ratio is 1:3 (DH 2011a).

People from BME backgrounds are less likely to access mental health services but are 40 per cent more likely to be referred to services through the criminal justice service (Commission for Healthcare Audit and Inspection 2007).

The Prison Reform Trust (2011) found that young offenders are more likely to experience mental health problems and drug and alcohol abuse in prison and are more likely to behave violently to others, to self-harm and to attempt suicide. They are more likely to report alcohol problems before going to prison than the general prison population (30%, compared to 19% of all prisoners).

Bullying and violence directed at prisoners, which can contribute to mental health problems, are now a major focus of HM Inspectorate of Prisons (HMIP), with the stated expectation that 'prisoners feel and are safe from victimisation from other prisoners and staff (which includes verbal and racial abuse, threats of violence and assault), through a clear and coordinated multidisciplinary approach' (HMIP 2012).

PEOPLE WITH LEARNING DISABILITIES

People with learning disabilities experience more discrimination than other people. They have a shorter life expectancy and are at risk of poorer general health because of increased likelihood of living in poverty, poor housing, being unemployed and experiencing discrimination (Emerson and Baines 2010). They are also more likely to suffer from mental health problems, including attention deficit hyperactivity disorder, personality disorders and behavioural disorders (Bernard and Turk 2009; Vanstraelen, Holt and Bouras 1997). Among the one in five children with recognized special educational needs (SEN), the prevalence rate of mental health disorders is estimated at 40 per cent at Key Stage 5 (ages 16–18 years), compared with 6 per cent of children without special needs (Meltzer et al. 2000).

Factors contributing to the psychological problems of children and adolescents with learning disabilities include the severity and cause of the learning disability and the presence of autistic spectrum disorder, and many social factors, including abuse and neglect, schooling issues, poverty and transgenerational social disadvantage. Hassles of daily living and parental psychiatric disorder also have serious effects (Bernard and Turk 2009).

Despite the high prevalence of mental disorders in children and young people with learning disabilities, they have particular problems in accessing appropriate mental health services. Child and Adolescent Mental Health Services generally lack the expertise required to assess and treat this group effectively. The negative impact this can have on families can lead to family breakdown and the need for expensive residential care (*ibid.*).

The association of mental health problems with learning disabilities continues into adulthood (Felce, Kerr and Hastings 2009). The *Independent Inquiry into Access to Healthcare for People with Learning Disabilities* (Michael 2008) found evidence that this group had higher levels of unmet need and received less effective care than the general population. Many reasons for this were identified, including a lack of awareness of the health needs of this group, poor training and education of clinical staff and negative attitudes of staff. People with learning disabilities are more likely to experience negative life events, such as abuse, harassment and violence (Knifton *et al.* 2010).

PEOPLE WITH LONG-TERM CONDITIONS OR PHYSICAL DISABILITY

People with long-term conditions or disability are the focus of Chapter 9, where we look at the impact of these physical conditions on mental health.

REFUGEES AND ASYLUM-SEEKERS

Two-thirds of refugees have experienced anxiety and depression. This may be linked to problems in their home countries (for instance, either witnessing or being the victim of war, rape, imprisonment or torture) (Mental Health Foundation 2007; NHS Greater Glasgow and Clyde 2013) or it may be because of social isolation or language difficulties or discrimination in their new country (Mental Health Foundation 2007). Post-traumatic stress disorder is a problem for many asylum-seekers (Rodger and Chappel 2008).

In leaving a country, families may be split, for example with one parent going ahead and the other to follow later with the children. As well as the disruption of any move, this brings the added burden of the psychological stress of separation (Tribe 2002). This particularly affects children, as mentioned in the earlier section on children and young people. The situation is even worse when a child is sent into exile unaccompanied (*ibid.*). There may be pre-existing mental health problems for which treatment cannot be obtained during the transition.

It can take many months for a refugee to receive a decision on refugee status. This causes stress and anxiety, with the asylum-seeker unable to plan for the future and still being afraid of being returned to their homeland. This can further adversely affect mental well-being (*ibid.*). If asylum-seekers are allowed to stay, it is quite likely that their socio-economic status will be lower than in their homeland (*ibid.*) and it may be difficult for them to find employment, so that they will experience economic deprivation and hardship, contributing to low self-esteem and mental ill health.

If a female refugee has undergone female genital mutilation (see Chapter 8) in her home country, migration can cause her to be more aware of its negative consequences (see the section on sexual abuse below), and some of these women may be ashamed to visit a doctor, particularly one who has not concealed their astonishment at the mutilation (Vloeberghs *et al.* 2012).

SEXUAL ABUSE AND SEXUAL EXPLOITATION

There is strong evidence of the effects of sexual abuse on children and the impact it has on adult mental health, resulting in higher rates of substance use, risky sexual behaviour and rates of sexually transmitted diseases (STDs) (Chartier, Walker and Naimark 2009; Friedman *et al.* 2011). Mullen *et al.* (1988) found that 20 per cent of women who had been abused as children had identifiable psychiatric disorders, mainly depressive, compared to 6 per cent of non-abused women.

Some groups are at particular risk of sexual abuse, such as foster children (Oswald, Heil and Goldbeck 2010), or children with physical or learning disabilities (National Working Group on Child Protection and Disability 2003). Female genital mutilation is discussed in our case study chapter on young BME groups.

Sexual exploitation, particularly of women and boys, has a serious impact on mental health. The Joseph Rowntree Foundation (Pearce, Williams and Galvin 2003) found high levels of self-harm, suicide or attempted suicide, regular heroin use and physical or sexual abuse (either as perpetrators or continuing as victims) in those who had been subjected to sexual abuse themselves.

Studies of sex offenders, including paedophiles, have found that their behaviour has been significantly influenced by adverse childhood experiences such as emotional or sexual abuse (Lee *et al.* 2002). Sexually victimized male adolescent sexual abusers are more likely than non-sexually victimized male adolescent abusers to have been exposed at an early age to pornography (Burton, Duty and Leibowitz 2011).

SEXUALITY

There is little robust evidence of the size or characteristics of the lesbian, gay, bisexual and transgender (LGBT) population (Aspinall 2009), nor of the prevalence of specific inequalities (Mitchell *et al.* 2008). This is due in part to a lack of understanding of the concept of sexual orientation, a lack of clear definitions, and difficulties with administering questions (Joloza *et al.* 2010). These problems are compounded by the concerns of the LGBT population in identifying themselves as such, given the harassment and discrimination many of them experience (Aspinall and Mitton 2008). Government estimates put the numbers of lesbian, gay and bisexual (LGB) people from 5 per cent to 7 per cent of the population (Shewell and Penn 2005). The size of the transgender population is even more difficult to estimate so cannot always be included as part of the LGBT group: their needs are in any case to do with identity rather than homosexuality. The Home Office identified rates from studies conducted in the Netherlands at between 1 in 11,900 and 1 in 17,000 men in the population. The ratio of female-to-male is much smaller than male-to-female, one estimate from Scotland being 1:4 (*ibid.*).

LGB people are more at risk of experiencing mental health problems than the population as a whole (DH 2007b).

Examples of issues in the LGBT community are:

- Bisexual people have poorer mental health than heterosexuals, gays or lesbians, with higher rates of anxiety, depression and suicidal thoughts (Dobinson *et al.* 2003).

- A total of 34 per cent of UK transgender people have attempted suicide (Kenagy 2005).

- The prevalence of mental disorders in LGB people is similar across ethnic groups (DH 2007a). However, in the UK, BME LGB people appear less likely to consider suicide, possibly because of cultural and religious taboos (National Working Group on Child Protection and Disability 2003), although young South Asian women are more at risk of self-harm and attempted suicide than white and African-Caribbean young women (DH 2007a).

- Young LGB people are four times more likely to experience depression than young people in general (McNamee 2006).

- Young gay and bisexual men are seven times more likely to have attempted suicide and three times more likely to have thought about killing themselves than their heterosexual counterparts (Remafedi *et al.* 1998).

- Gay and bisexual men are more than five times more likely than heterosexual men to self-harm and lesbian and bisexual women twice as likely (Skeg *et al.* 2003). Bisexual people are more likely to self-harm than lesbians or gays (Bennett 2004).

Good mental health is associated with high self-esteem. Gay men and lesbians are more likely than their bisexual peers to be 'out' to their family and to health professionals (DH 2007b), and family acceptance of young LGBT people is associated with positive mental health (Ryan *et al.* 2010).

Poor mental health is associated with experiences of victimization and perceived discrimination (Mays and Cochran 2001). Those in the LGBT population with mental health problems are more likely to report ongoing discrimination than heterosexual people:

- Bisexual people and gay men are more likely to report to having lost their job as a consequence of discrimination (DH 2007b). (See section in Chapter 2 on unemployment and its effects on mental health.)
- Lesbians report more verbal and physical abuse than heterosexual women (National Working Group on Child Protection and Disability 2003).
- LGB people are more likely to self-harm as a consequence of discrimination (Meyer 2003).
- The LGBT population are more at risk of sexual abuse than the heterosexual population (Cramer, McNiel and Holley 2012).

LGB people use mental health services more often than the heterosexual population, but one-third of gay men, a quarter of bisexual men and more than 40 per cent of lesbians have more negative experiences. In one in five cases, mental health professionals may make a causal link between a person's mental health issue and their sexual orientation. Experiences range from lack of empathy to homophobic incidents (National Working Group on Child Protection and Disability 2003). This has implications for the need for training for health care professionals (Rutherford *et al.* 2012).

SOCIAL ISOLATION AND INCLUSION

Social issolation, which older people are especially vulnerable to (as discussed further under lifespan in Chapter 4) is recognized by the government as a major issue for mental health, perhaps the most significant factor after income and poverty (NIMHE 2005). Social isolation can involve a great many distressing feelings, such as powerlessness, alienation, meaninglessness and self-estrangement. It is often associated with loneliness, although the two concepts differ, with social isolation being the objective state of deprivation of social contact and loneliness the experience of subjective feelings (Biordi and Nicholson 2013).

The groups most at risk of social isolation tend to be those we already recognize as needing added support, such as older people, minority ethnic populations, the homeless and those living in poverty. However, throughout the life course, other groups also suffer from loneliness.

Children are reporting more experiences of loneliness than in previous years. In 2008/2009, ChildLine counselled more than 5500 children with loneliness, sadness and isolation as their main problem and almost 4400 children with loneliness as an additional problem (NSPCC 2010). The top problems associated with their loneliness were family relationship problems, bullying and physical abuse. Depression, mental health problems, school problems and bereavement were also associated with loneliness (*ibid.*). Teenagers are believed to be especially vulnerable to loneliness because their brains are still developing, so they may 'misread social cues and other people's emotions' (Mental Health Foundation 2010c, p.14). People in middle age are exposed to various risks for loneliness, including changes to the family when children leave home, bereavement, divorce or retirement (Mental Health Foundation 2012).

There is a clear relationship between social support and the risk of mortality and morbidity (APHO 2007; Berkman and Kawachi 2000). People with few social contacts are at increased risk of mental health problems (Stewart-Brown 2002). Social networks can prevent problems arising from stress, and research suggests that they can help women recover from depression (Brugha *et al.* 1990) and reduce the risk of depression (Morgan and Swann 2004).

The most common measure of perceived support is whether or not an individual has a confiding and close relationship with a significant other (Cooper *et al.* 1999). However, it needs to be recognized that the support provided within relationships varies enormously. Marriage, a critical significant relationship, can be fraught with difficulties, including lack of support, as well as the undermining and destructive effects of domestic violence (Fletcher and Kerr 2010).

Those in paid work and those in higher socio-economic groups have been found to have larger networks and greater participation and perceived support. People *feel* busier today than 30 years ago, but unemployed people, who may be assumed to have more time, are less likely to be engaged in social groups. Women who work part time participate to a greater extent (Skocpol 1996).

Ethnic minorities are at increased risk of the poor health consequences of the lack of social networks. However, it appears that those in a minority group have better mental health if they live in areas where a greater proportion of the population come from the same minority group, be it race, religion or occupation based (Halpern 1993).

High levels of stress are associated with low social support; social isolation is common among depressed patients (Morgan and Swann 2004). Social support may improve mental health by offering opportunities for social interaction and help with practical problems, thus reducing loneliness, enhancing self-esteem and feelings of self-worth, and improving levels of perceived support (Cooper *et al.* 1999, p.15).

As well as social exclusion contributing to mental ill health, people with mental health problems face particular problems of exclusion. The government document *Mental Health and Social Exclusion* (Social Exclusion Unit 2004) identified five main reasons for this:

- Stigma and discrimination against people who have mental health problems.
- Low expectations of professionals as to what those with mental health problems can achieve.
- Lack of clear responsibility for promotion of positive outcomes for those with mental health problems, in terms of employment and social opportunities.
- Lack of ongoing support to enable people to work.
- Barriers to engaging in the community, including poor access to decent housing, transport, education, arts and leisure facilities.

VETERANS OF THE ARMED SERVICES

There are an estimated five million veterans (people who have served with the armed forces) in the UK, with a further 20,000 people leaving the armed forces each year (NHS Choices 2012b). In 2010, 164 personnel were discharged from the forces as a consequence of mental health problems, 21 per cent of them with post-traumatic stress disorder. Annually, approximately 1 in 1000 personnel have to leave for mental health reasons. It has been estimated that just over 27 per cent of veterans experience a common mental health problem, and those under the age of 24 years have been found to be two to three times more at risk of suicide than their contemporaries in the general population (Kapur *et al.* 2009).

The UK Government does not record suicides among ex-soldiers, so numbers can be hard to obtain. However, the BBC's *Panorama* programme (BBC 2013b), via a Freedom of Information (FoI) request to the Ministry of Defence (MoD), found that 21 serving soldiers and 29 veterans took their own lives in 2012, more than were killed in action.

For some ex-servicemen or women, returning to civilian life can be difficult. The military can provide a supportive structure, including comradeship and friendship. Transition into the general community can put pressure on important relationships, particularly married partners, which can lead to mental distress (NHS Confederation 2010). Veterans experiencing mental health problems are reluctant to access support or treatment, often not coming forward until an average of 14 years have passed since their discharge (*ibid.*). This may be due partly to the stigma that ex-service personnel experience from the general population (Murrison 2010). It may also be a consequence of veterans underestimating the difficulties of adjusting to civilian life and the critical need for social networks (Johnson and Johnson 2011).

Associated with mental health problems within the armed forces is that of alcohol abuse. This is more common in veterans who have been in combat (Fear *et al.* 2010). It has been estimated that about 18 per cent of veterans have an alcohol-related problem (Johnson and Johnson 2011). Some of this may be related to the culture of heavy drinking found in some military units (NHS Confederation 2010).

Veterans are more likely than the general population to experience social exclusion, homelessness and crime, all of which are associated with mental illness (Johnsen, Jones and Rugg 2008). It was estimated in 2007 by the Sir Oswald Stoll Foundation that one in ten homeless people is a veteran, with a similar number being in prison (Mental Health Foundation 2010a).

VICTIMS AND SURVIVORS OF DOMESTIC VIOLENCE

Domestic violence accounts for 16–25 per cent of all recorded violent crime (DCLG 2010). Women sometimes do not report domestic violence as a consequence of fear of not being believed and/or being humiliated (MoJ 2010). The British Crime Survey (Jansson 2007) found that 34 per cent of the women and 62 per cent of the men who reported that they had suffered domestic violence since the age of 16 years had probably never told anyone other than the survey. This means that estimated figures are probably underestimates.

Of the estimated two million victims of domestic abuse in England and Wales in 2011/2012, 1.2 million were women (ONS 2013b). Men are much less likely to report themselves as victims of domestic violence, but it is estimated that one in five men experience domestic violence (compared to one in four women) (BMA 2007).

Domestic violence can have both short-term and long-term effects on physical and mental health, leading to acute and chronic physical injury, loss of hearing and vision, physical disfigurement, depression, alcoholism and sometimes suicide (Abbott and Williamson 1999). Women experiencing domestic violence are more likely to abuse alcohol or drugs, to attempt suicide and be diagnosed with depression or psychosis (Stark *et al.* 1981). It is estimated that two women a week die from domestic violence incidents in Britain (Mirrlees-Black 1999).

Domestic violence has potentially devastating consequences for children. Children's educational attainment is adversely affected and they may have limited social skills, exhibit violent, risky or disruptive behaviour or suffer from depression or severe anxiety (UNICEF 2006). Children who grow up in violent homes are also more likely to be victims of child abuse and grow up to become victims or perpetrators as adults (*ibid.*). Domestic violence in the antenatal period is associated with high rates of antenatal and post-natal depression, which is linked to behavioural problems in the child at 3–4 years (Flach *et al.* 2011).

Groups particularly vulnerable to domestic violence include:

- Older people, mainly in the form of neglect (Lees 2000); up to 4 per cent of older people living at home with their partners/family as carers are abused (O'Keefe *et al.* 2007).

- Pregnant women – 30 per cent of cases begin during pregnancy (Walby and Allen 2004) and domestic violence is a prime cause of miscarriage or stillbirth (Mezey 1997) and of maternal deaths during childbirth (Lewis and Drife 2004); contributory factors are: pregnancy being unintended, lower economic status, and being unmarried (James, Brody and Hamilton 2013).

- Women fleeing violence – they are at greatest risk of homicide at the point of separation or after leaving a violent partner (Lees 2000).

- Some Asian families in which it may be more common to tolerate abuse; forced marriage is also recognized as a form of domestic violence (Walby and Allen 2004).

Domestic violence can also contribute to homelessness, either because a partner flees from the home or because of eviction following unacceptable behaviour. The contribution of homelessness to mental ill health was discussed earlier.

PRINCIPLES INTO PRACTICE

This chapter has focused on the first two of our underlying principles: mental health and well-being is a holistic concept, and it is vital to address the social, economic, political, cultural and environmental factors that enhance mental health and well-being through a consideration of a wide range of life circumstances that impact on them. It has also used the third principle of identifying need in specific sections of the population. Finally, with respect to the fourth principle, involving communities, users and carers in setting priorities, the importance of carers is highlighted.

Chapter 4

WHAT AFFECTS MENTAL HEALTH AND WELL-BEING?

INDIVIDUAL LIFE STAGE AND PERSONAL BEHAVIOURS

KEY POINTS

Throughout the course of life, many different factors can affect mental health and well-being and problems can have wide-reaching effects:

- Young people's mental health is affected by parenting, deprivation, education and bullying.
- Depression affects 13 per cent of mothers, and psychiatric disorders are the main cause of maternal death.
- Working-age adults have significant levels of mental ill health, with wide-ranging impacts on families, workplaces and communities.
- In older people, physical ill health contributes to mental ill health. Social isolation is also significant.
- Terminal illness affects the emotional health of carers and families as well as that of the patient.
- Personal behaviours contribute to mental health and well-being.
- Healthy eating can improve both physical and mental health.
- Physical activity is beneficial to both physical and mental well-being.

- There are strong links between poor mental health and smoking, drinking alcohol and substance misuse.
- Mental health is adversely affected by many factors but it also influences many of them. For example, physical ill health and unhealthy eating increase the risk of mental ill health, but those with mental ill health are less likely to participate in physical exercise or to eat healthily.
- Access to health improvement services for people with mental health problems is critical and often not done very well.

INTRODUCTION

This chapter continues to consider the distribution of mental health, mental illness and well-being. Here we focus on individual factors, particularly as they change during the life course. Genetic predisposition and gender issues are also discussed where relevant. The second half of the chapter goes on to describe the way in which personal lifestyle behaviour impacts on mental health and well-being (and vice versa).

ACROSS THE LIFESPAN

A 'lifespan' approach to mental health and well-being was developed by Cattan and Tilford (2006) from work with students wanting a framework with which they could identify in their working lives, often with specific population groups. Using this lifespan approach, the following subsections look at mental health issues chronologically for people in six major life stages: children and young people, adolescents, antenatal and post-natal women and parenting, working-age adults, older people and people at the end of life.

Children and young people

Estimates suggest that almost a quarter of the UK's population of approximately 63 million people is under 20 years old, fairly evenly split among the following age groups: under 5 years of age, 5–9 years, 10–14 years and 15–19 years (ONS 2012a). Childhood is a formative stage: the impacts on cognitive abilities happen at a very young age (Marmot 2010b).

An extensive ONS report (Meltzer *et al.* 2000) found that about 11 per cent of boys and 8 per cent of girls in the UK aged from 5 to 15 years had a mental health problem, most commonly emotional disorders (depression, anxiety and phobias), hyperactivity (inattention and over-activity) and conduct disorders (difficult, aggressive and antisocial behaviour). With age, the rates for all conditions increase: approximately 8 per cent of children aged 5–10 years and 12 per cent of children aged 11–15 years have a mental health problem. The highest rates were found in Black children (12%) and the lowest in Indian children (4%). Prevalence rates of mental disorders have been found to be greater among children in certain family circumstances. For example: 16 per cent of children in lone-parent families have a mental disorder compared to 8 per cent of those in a two-parent family; 15 per cent of children in reconstituted families compared to 9 per cent with no step-children; 18 per cent of those in families with more than four children compared with 8 per cent of those with two; 20 per cent of those with both parents unemployed compared to 8 per cent with two parents working; and 14 per cent of those in families in social class V compared with 5 per cent in social class I[3] (*ibid.*).

The importance of a mother or primary 'attachment figure' for a child in its first two years has been stressed by many writers, following the influential work of John Bowlby, who suggested that the long-term consequences of lacking this figure may include depression and increased aggression (McLeod 2007).

There is a strong relationship between poor physical health and mental health problems (Kim *et al.* 2012). Meltzer *et al.* (2000) found that the proportion of children with poor physical health was 6 per cent, but 20 per cent of those also suffered from a mental disorder. The most common associated problems were: bedwetting (12% of those with a mental health problem compared with 4% without), speech or language problems (12% compared with 3%), coordination difficulties (8% compared with 2%) and soiling (4% compared with 1%).

---

3   Social classes I–V are defined by Meltzer *et al.* as: I) professionals; II) managerial and technical; III) skilled occupations (manual and non-manual); IV) partly skilled occupations and V) unskilled occupations.

Children with poor school attendance are less likely to succeed academically and are more likely not to be in education, employment or training when they leave school (Taylor 2012). In England's state-funded primary and secondary schools in the autumn term of 2012, 0.9 per cent of pupils (more than 53,000) were persistent absentees (having missed 46 or more sessions) and almost 400,000 pupils (6.4%) were at risk of becoming persistent absentees (having missed 22 or more sessions, (DfE 2013). There is also a direct link between school absenteeism and a higher prevalence of mental health problems in adolescence (BPS 2012).

Poor mental health in childhood is strongly associated with both poor physical health in adulthood (Goodwin *et al.* 2009) and poor mental health in adulthood, the latter particularly in males (Clark *et al.* 2007). Conduct problems are associated with various poor outcomes, including parenthood at a young age, criminal activity, unemployment, substance abuse, divorce or separation and psychiatric disorders (Beecham *et al.* 2011). Premature mortality is also associated with early problem behaviours, as a consequence of the increased likelihood of poor health-related habits, including earlier and higher rates of smoking and binge-drinking (Von Stumm *et al.* 2011).

Good mental health provides considerable protection against becoming involved in unhealthy behaviours. The early family situation that a child experiences, in terms of material circumstances and interpersonal relationships and interactions, is a key influence throughout the life course. Sources of resilience include social support from adults (such as grandparents), parental bahaviour that encourages self-esteem, breastfeeding and a learning environment in the home (Friedli 2009).

According to the Children's Society's measures, half a million children in the UK are unhappy (Rees *et al.* 2012). The Children's Society (2012) suggests that interventions to improve this should focus on specific approaches, such as providing an environment that encourages learning and development and promotes good self-esteem; providing a safe home and local environment; and presenting opportunities to become involved in positive activities.

Adolescents

Many of the issues around mental health and well-being in adolescents[4] continue to be the same as those in children and young people (including, for example, bullying), while some are common to adolescents and adults (including, for example, problems with alcohol). However, some aspects are specific to adolescents and some conditions may begin in adolescence, such as social anxiety disorder (one of the most persistent anxiety disorders) with a median age of onset of 13 years (NICE 2013a).

Risk taking among adolescents is a key concern for health professionals, and most morbidity in this age group is related to drug and alcohol misuse, tobacco use, sexual behaviour, poor diet and physical inactivity. Each of these is discussed further in the section looking at personal behaviours.

Mental well-being in earlier life appears to be related to mental well-being later in life. In a longitudinal study, Richard and Huppert (2011) found that adolescents with positive well-being were found to have a low likelihood of emotional problems, to have a high satisfaction with work, high contact rates with friends and family and to engage in social activities in mid-life.

Patterns of mental health in adolescence vary by sex:

- Girls self-harm almost four times as much as boys (WHEC 2013).

- Young women are twice as likely as young men to suffer a depressive disorder (*ibid.*).

- Girls appear to have lower levels of life satisfaction than boys, and to worry more than boys (AYPH 2011).

- Girls' disengagement from school is often a hidden and invisible problem (WHEC 2013).

- Teenage mothers are three times more likely to develop post-natal depression and other mental health problems than older mothers (CAMHS Review 2008).

- The rate at which young women are drinking heavily has increased dramatically in the last ten years: half of 15 year-old girls reported being drunk in the past week (compared with 37%

4   'Adolescence' means turning from a child to an adult. There is no fixed age range, although the term 'adult' in the UK is usually classed as starting at 18, or sometimes 16, and children's services sometimes cover up to age 16.

of boys). Heavy drinking puts women at risk of accidents and makes them vulnerable to assault. A figure of 12 per cent of girls reported having unprotected sex after drinking alcohol (WHEC 2013, p.17).

Antenatal and post-natal women and parenting

There are significant issues around mental well-being for women both before and after they give birth. While they are vulnerable to the same range of mental health disorders as other adults, some problems are exacerbated:

- Some disorders may worsen, e.g. bipolar disorder (Jones and Craddock 2005).

- Disorders may need more urgent intervention because of risk to the foetus and the effect on women's physical health and care (NICE 2007).

- Post-natal-onset psychotic disorders may be severe (Ryan and Kostaras 2005).

- Use of illicit drugs in pregnancy and breastfeeding (Economidoy, Klimi and Vivilaki 2012; Friguls et al. 2010).

There is little evidence that pre-existing disorders change during this time, with the exception of bipolar disorder. Nor is there much evidence that the prognoses of disorders that develop in this period are significantly different from those developing at other times (Brockington 1996). However, a mental disorder in a pregnant woman (even a condition such as anxiety, which is often considered a mild mental health problem) can have a significant effect on the well-being of the woman, foetus and infant (NICE 2007). Severe depression is associated with stillbirth, obstetric complications and low birth weight infants (Bonari et al. 2004; Lobel, Dunkel-Schetter and Scrimshaw 1992; Lou et al. 1994; Wadhwa et al. 1993). Women with bipolar disorder or schizophrenia are at increased risk of pre-term delivery (Lewis and Drife 2004) and low birth weight infants (Howard 2005). Maternal psychoses appear to increase the risk of stillbirth (Webb et al. 2005). The relationship with the partner may also suffer, and mental illness may increase the risk to the partner's mental health (Lovestone and Kumar 1993).

Depression affects about 13 per cent of mothers (O'Hara and Swain 1996). For some, recovery is spontaneous, within six months. For others, it may last months, even years, if untreated, and recur over time or with the birth of another baby (Cox 1989). Obsessive compulsive disorder (OCD) is much more common in women who had post-natal depression than in those who did not (41% versus 6%) (Abramowitz et al. 2003).

Identified risk factors for depression in the post-natal period include:

- psychiatric history (NCCMH 2007)
- depressed mood or anxiety during pregnancy (Elliott et al. 2000)
- poor levels of social support, both emotional (having partner, friends and family) and instrumental (practical help) (Robertson, Jones and Haque 2004)
- older age – older mothers, aged from 40 to 44 years, have been found to be five times as likely to have been depressed as younger women (Mental Health Foundation 2012).

Poor or untreated maternal mental illness may also contribute to poorer long-term outcomes, such as cognitive delay, emotional and behavioural difficulties in young children (Nulman et al. 2002), parenting difficulties and poor mental health outcomes for children (Beardslee, Bemporad and Keller 1983; Kuosmanen et al. 2010). Children affected may then continue to have psychological problems in adulthood (Green et al. 2005).

Several studies have shown the importance of breastfeeding not just for physical reasons but also for the emotional well-being of both mother and baby, in terms of bonding (Bick et al. 2002). Health services have a role to play in encouraging breastfeeding.

Failings in services for different groups of women have been identified: women in disadvantaged areas do not receive the same quality of care, which impacts on their and their children's health (DH 2009b). It has also been argued that not enough attention is paid to women's own experiences of pregnancy and delivery, including childbirth-related post-traumatic stress disorder, perinatal bereavement and parent-to-infant attachment disorders (Condon 2010). These are relatively common and would benefit from identification and treatment for mother, infant and family as a whole.

Working-age adults

Mental health issues related to employment status were discussed in Chapter 2. This subsection looks at issues affecting adults, generally before they are likely to experience problems more associated with older age.

As Dame Carol Black (2008, p.4) pointed out, people of working age are 'individuals whose health has consequences often far beyond themselves – touching their families and children, workplaces and wider communities'. Self-esteem and self-belief are crucial to all decisions an adult takes regarding relationships, work, parenting and social interaction.

Among women in England, the peak age for common mental disorders is 45–54 (25%); in men the peak age is 25–54 (15%) (NHSIC 2009). Five million people of working age have a common mental health disorder and just under a million have a severe condition (Gillborn 2008). Mental health conditions are probably undiagnosed to a greater extent than other conditions in this age group, as their presence can affect an individual's position in the workplace and lead to discrimination (as discussed earlier).

There are several important differences among working-age population groups in the prevalence of mental health conditions. For example, women tend to experience poorer mental health than men:

- A total of 63 per cent of women have experienced some form of low-level mental health problem in their lifetime (WHEC 2013, p.17).
- Women in England were more likely than men to have a common mental disorder (20% and 13% respectively), and rates were significantly higher for women across all categories of common mental disorder with the exception of panic disorder and obsessive compulsive disorder (NHSIC 2009).
- Women are twice as likely to become depressed as men and more likely to experience depression for longer periods of time (WHEC 2013).
- The overall prevalence of psychotic disorder in the past year was 0.4 per cent (0.3% of men, 0.5% of women). In both men and women the highest prevalence was observed in those aged 35 to 44 years (0.7% and 1.1% respectively) (NHSIC 2009).

Although women are more likely to have been treated for a mental health problem than men (29% as compared to 17%), it is believed this may be because women are more likely to report symptoms of common mental health problems (Mental Health Foundation n.d. b). Depression may be under-reported in men because they present to the GP with different symptoms. There are some problems more common in men:

- Men are more likely than women to have alcohol and drug problems (Mental Health Foundation 2007).
- All personality disorders are more prevalent in men, apart from the schizotypal category. Men are five times more likely than women to be diagnosed with antisocial personality disorder (*ibid.*).

Older people

Nationally, life expectancy has increased dramatically in recent decades: by 2035, life expectancy at birth is projected to reach 83.4 years for men and 87 years for women (ONS 2011a). The number of older people is increasing: it is estimated that in 2035 in the UK there will be 30 million people aged more than 60 years (compared to 19 million in 2010), of whom 3.5 million will be 85 years or over (compared to 1.4 million in 2010) (ONS 2011b).

Positive mental and emotional health and well-being is as important to older people as it is at any other time of life, even though there is an assumption that depression is a 'normal' aspect of ageing (Mental Health Foundation 2011). There are differences in estimates of the prevalence of mental health problems in older people but they appear less likely to have a neurotic disorder (or common mental health problem), other than depression, than other sections of the British population (Mental Health Foundation 2007).

ONS figures suggest:

- a figure of 12 per cent of older women and 8 per cent of older men have a significant level of reported neurotic symptoms
- up to 5 per cent of men and 10 per cent of women over the age of 65 are being treated for depression, which is the commonest mental disorder in old age

- the prevalence of common mental disorder – depression, anxiety, phobias – decreases with age, particularly for men until the age of about 85. Before this age, older people actually have better mental health than the population on average.

(Evans *et al.* 2003)

However, research findings are mixed and Taylor *et al.* (2007) found ageing to be associated with an increased prevalence of mental disorders. They estimated that 40 per cent of older people seeing their GP may have a mental health disorder but only one-third will have discussed depression with the GP. Age Concern (2007) estimated that 3 million older people in the UK experience mental health problems, of whom 25 per cent have symptoms of depression and 10–15 per cent are clinically depressed.

Depression in older people can be triggered by particular life events (Brooker and Surr 2005), including the onset of poor physical health, retirement, bereavement, divorce, illness of partner and becoming a carer (Allen 2008). Other risk factors include social isolation, alcohol abuse and family history or previous episodes of depression (Nicholls 2006). Two in five people over the age of 65 living in care homes suffer from depression, twice the rate of those living in the community (Mental Health Foundation 2007).

Alcohol abuse in old age is often unrecognized, despite approximately 20 per cent of older men and just more than 7 per cent of older women drinking at levels that could be harmful for their health. Of these, up to 30 per cent become depressed and are at increased risk of suicide. Other problems associated with alcohol abuse include anxiety, hearing voices, confusion and dementia. The lack of recognition of alcohol problems increases the risk associated with taking medication at the same time (Mental Health Foundation 2011). (See also later section on personal behaviours.)

An estimated 70 per cent of new cases of depression in older people are related to poor physical health (Mental Health Foundation 2007). Social isolation in older people has been linked with increased mortality rates and a range of poor health outcomes, including cardiovascular disease (Sorkin, Rook and Lu 2002). For all age groups, physical activity is associated with better mental health, but older people are least likely to partake in appropriate levels of exercise (Allen 2008). It has been shown that those who do participate in exercise experience improved mood and better self-perceptions of health (Fox *et al.* 2007).

Up to 17 per cent of people aged more than 64 years may be socially isolated (having an absence of contact with other people, measured through frequency of contact with family and friends) (Hawton *et al.* 2011). Social isolation can be a particular problem for older men, too, especially for those who are widowed or divorced and who may have relied on partners to organize their social life and maintain contact with families. The resulting problem is compounded as they may present to the GP with a physical problem, while the underlying problem is a mental health problem such as depression (Mental Health Foundation 2010b). (Social isolation was also discussed in Chapter 3.)

Many factors can prevent older people fully participating in an active social life, such as difficulties with physical access and limited transport. The over-60s are at the lowest risk of crime, but fear of crime can be a significant deterrent to going out of the house. Actually being a victim of crime can have a significant and long-lasting effect on older people's well-being, in some cases leading to serious depression and withdrawal from social engagement (ONS 2008).

Dementia can be a further reason for older people not participating fully. About 800,000 people in the UK have dementia, and the numbers are forecast to double by 2040 (DH 2013c). Poor mental health is associated with dementia, especially anxiety (which is linked to depression). Psychosis can often accompany dementia, particularly delusions of persecution, agitation and aggression (Shub and Kunik 2009).

Older people are more likely to be involved in religious activity, and this seems to be related to less depression and anxiety, greater reported quality of life and less cognitive impairment (Luanaigh and Lawlor 2008). This may be as a consequence of the increased social opportunities that religious organizations offer, as well as the meaning and purpose that people derive from their beliefs.

End of life

The quality of the end of life experience is crucial for the individual concerned, and for those close to them. It is also an issue in terms of use of health and social care resources. Some people die as they would have wished, but many do not receive quality care at the end of their lives. For many, a 'good death' would involve not only being free from pain but being treated with respect and dignity, in famiiar surroundings in the company of friends or family (DH 2008).

People are uncomfortable talking about dying and death, so that when they come to the end of their lives friends and loved ones are not aware of their preferences (*ibid.*). A major mismatch has been identified between people's preferences for where they would like to die and their actual place of death: about 70 per cent of people would prefer to die at home, yet currently about 60 per cent die in hospital (Dying Matters n.d.).

Estimates suggest that there are more than 49,000 children and young people in the UK with life-threatening conditions that may need palliative care (helping people to deal with their illness or condition – for instance, with pain control and psychological or social support – without curing it). Such cases have significant effects on the emotional health of the whole family (Together for Short Lives 2012). Children face many of the difficulties faced by adults but may also be afraid and suffering from misunderstanding or lack of knowledge (*ibid.*), which increases anxiety and will adversely affect their emotional well-being.

There are emotional as well as practical issues not only for those who are dying but for those who will be left behind. Particularly affected may be parents and siblings of children who have died, children whose parents have died and those who have been caring for the deceased. Depression is common in these groups, as discussed in the previous chapter.

PERSONAL BEHAVIOURS

In this section we consider the effects of personal behaviours, the way in which someone's lifestyle choices can also influence their mental health and well-being. It is recognized that these choices are made in the context of the social and environmental conditions described in Chapter 2 and the circumstances described in Chapter 3 and should not be considered in isolation.

The sequence of behaviours considered starts with the two that affect everybody (eating and physical activity), and then goes on to those related to use and misuse of substances, followed by sexual health and finally the effect of suicide on those involved.

Healthy eating

Eating well is important in ensuring good physical health, and there is increasing evidence of links between diet and mental health or ill health (Swanton 2008). Poor diet can affect feelings of general well-being, because the lack of essential nutrients (particularly essential fatty acids, antioxidants and minerals in fruit and vegetables) can reduce levels of energy, lessen the ability to fight off infections and lead to mood changes. Several large studies have linked low intake of particular nutrients (most significantly folate and folic acid but also zinc and vitamins B1, B2 and C) with higher levels of depression (Cornah 2004).

Changing farming techniques (including the use of pesticides and the increase in fats in meat) are sometimes implicated in poor mental health, as are increasingly refined, processed foods, and the introduction of increasing numbers of additives (*ibid.*). Food produced in this way tends to be high in fat and sugar content, contributing to an increase in obesity (Butland *et al.* 2007).

The numbers classed as obese or overweight has been increasing rapidly since the 1980s. An estimated one in four adults and one in five children aged 10 or 11 in the UK are obese (NHS Choices 2012a). Obesity is considerably more common in those on low income compared to those on high incomes (Prescott-Clarke and Primatesta 1998), as is poor mental health.

Being overweight can have a major impact on a person's confidence and feeling of well-being (Polivy 1996). Scott *et al.* (2008) found significant associations between obesity and both depression and anxiety. This association can work in either direction: people who are depressed or anxious gain weight from eating. Changed eating habits are an indicator of depression (NCCMH 2004a). Also, an obese person is less likely to engage in physical exercise, so missing out on the advantages it may have in improving their mental as well as physical well-being (see following subsection).

In addition to the psychological aspects of being overweight, some anti-obesity drugs can lead to depression. For example, rimonabant is associated with increasing the chances of depression and suicidal thoughts (NHS Knowledge Services 2007). Drugs prescribed for mental illness can also lead to obesity (Rethink 2004).

Other food-related mental health problems include eating disorders. These comprise a number of conditions that affect the way people consume food, and have physical, psychological and social implications. The Adult Psychiatric Morbidity Survey (NHSIC 2009) found that in England 9 per cent of women and 4 per cent of men had had a possible eating disorder in the past year. The prevalence decreased with age, and this was particularly pronounced for women (20% of women aged 16–24 compared with 1% aged 75 and over).

The most common eating disorders are:

- anorexia nervosa, when someone tries to keep their weight low, by not eating or by exercising excessively
- bulimia, when someone binge eats and then deliberately makes themselves sick or uses laxatives to control their weight
- binge eating, when someone has a compulsion to overeat.

(NCCMH 2004b)

Eating disorders cause extreme distress to both the individuals and their families, and they need treatment, as they can be life-threatening. NICE (2004b) recommends a full assessment and a range of treatments, initially in the community, including self-help, through to hospital admission where necessary.

Physical activity

The importance of an active lifestyle in maintaining and improving physical health has been recognized for decades. There is also extensive evidence that physical activity is effective in preventing mental ill health (particularly anxiety and depression), improving the quality of life for people with mental illness and as a treatment for mild to moderate depression (APHO 2007; Biddle 2000; Halliwell 2005; Mead *et al.* 2009; Whitelaw *et al.* 2008). Harvey *et al.* (2010) found that leisure-time physical exercise (specifically leisure-time rather than workplace activity) reduced symptoms of depression and that the effects were related not to the intensity of the activity, but to the higher levels of social engagement and social support people received when participating in physical activity. Exercise may act as a diversionary approach to negative thoughts. It may also have physiological effects such as changes in endorphin and monoamine levels (NCCMH 2011c).

Alcohol

Deaths caused by the consumption of alcohol have doubled over the past 20 years in the UK. Increasingly, it is younger people who are affected. Dangerous drinking is closely associated with living in areas of high deprivation, where the rates of alcohol-related deaths are approximately 45 per cent higher than average (Breakwell *et al.* 2007).

The Adult Psychiatric Morbidity Survey (NHSIC 2009) found that 33 per cent of men and 16 per cent of women in England's adult population living in private households were drinking at hazardous levels. However, prevalence decreased markedly with age. The peak of women's drinking was 16–24 years (32% drinking hazardously), whereas it was 25–34 years for men (46%). There was some degree of alcohol dependence in 8.7 per cent of men and 3.3 per cent of women.

Many studies (e.g. Evans *et al.* 2003) have shown the close relationship between poor mental health and alcohol problems. The Institute of Alcohol Studies (IAS 2007) identifies the complexity of this relationship: mental health problems and alcohol problems can be causally linked either way; genetics or early family environment could contribute to either problem; there might be some positive effects of light to moderate drinking on mental health for some; and heavy drinking might lead to misuse of other substances, which then has a further adverse impact on mental health.

Almost all drinkers seeking help for their problem report symptoms of anxiety and depression. Research is inconclusive about whether drinking causes depression, but its impact on personal circumstances, such as unemployment or relationship breakdown, along with feelings of hopelessness and guilt, may exacerbate the likelihood of anxiety and depression (Alcohol Concern n.d.). Heavy and binge drinking by young people can be a mechanism for coping with stress or anxiety (Newbury-Birch *et al.* 2008).

Research suggests that alcohol misuse among young people is a major risk factor in the development of mental health problems. Adverse consequences include side effects (such as headaches, sleep disturbance and appetite changes), effects on cognitive function and memory, depression, stress and anxiety, poor school performance, and difficulties in maintaining friendships.

Newbury-Birch *et al.* (2009) found evidence for the following risks associated with children, young people and alcohol:

- genetic history
- childhood abuse
- early contact with alcohol consumption, often through family members
- past family history of alcohol abuse
- behavioural problems of child/young person which may be predictive of alcohol problems, such as antisocial behaviour, sensation-seeking or impulsive personality types.

It has been generally accepted that alcohol consumption declines with age, as a consequence of changes in life circumstances, attitudes and increasing ill health. However, there is now evidence that the older population today drink more heavily than previously, because of higher levels of disposable income and increased availability and acceptability of alcohol. This is of particular concern given that tolerance to alcohol is significantly lowered in the elderly (IAS 2010). This may have an appreciable effect on the mental health of older people.

Smoking

Although smoking rates are declining, about 22 per cent of adult men and 21 per cent of adult women are smokers, with the highest rate being among younger women (31% of 20–24 year-old women) and slightly older men (30% of 25–34 year-old men) (ASH 2011b).

People with poor mental health are significantly more likely to smoke and have higher levels of nicotine dependency. Psychiatric patients are two to three times more likely to smoke than the general population, with 40–50 per cent of people with depression and anxiety disorders, and 70 per cent of people with severe mental illness (such as schizophrenia), smoking (Olivier, Lubman and Fraser 2007).

Not only do people who have a mental health disorder smoke more, but people who smoke are more at risk of developing a mental health problem, including being prone to higher suicide rates (FPH 2008). A causal relationship has not been established, but some studies suggest that smoking could act as a trigger for the development of mental health problems (West and Jarvis 2005).

The many reasons for high levels of smoking in people with a mental health problem include attempted self-medication of symptoms of depression and anxiety and using smoking as a coping mechanism (ASH 2011b).

High levels of smoking significantly contribute to the physical ill health and mortality of people with mental health disorders. People with schizophrenia or bipolar depression are almost twice as likely to die from coronary heart disease (CHD) and four times more likely to die from respiratory disease than the general population (DH 2006b). Smoking is a key causal factor in these diseases (ASH 2011a).

The physical benefits of stopping smoking are numerous but, additionally, ex-smokers overwhelmingly report being happier for having given up smoking (Shahab and West 2009).

Illicit drug use

Two million people in the UK smoke cannabis and half of all 16–29 year-olds have tried it at least once (RCPsych 2009). Several major studies have shown that people who use cannabis are more likely to develop schizophrenia, particularly the younger the age of smoking it (*ibid.*). It is unclear as to whether cannabis causes mental health disorders or that people with these disorders use it as a medication. One study of school children aged 14–15 years found that those who used cannabis were significantly more likely to suffer from depression, but not vice versa – young people with depression were no more likely than others to use cannabis (Patton *et al.* 2002).

Cocaine, when taken in small amounts, causes euphoria and a feeling of being mentally alert, talkative and energetic. However, repeated exposure leads to adaptation, wherein the user becomes tolerant and potentially addicted. In the long term, cocaine use can lead to increasing restlessness, irritability, panic attacks and paranoia, and even full-blown psychosis (National Institute on Drug Abuse 2010).

The instant effects of taking heroin are pleasure, relief of pain and drowsiness. There is a risk of death as a result of overdose. Symptoms of anxiety and depression are likely to increase. Hallucinations can be stronger with people who have a history of psychosis, and heroin can interfere with psychiatric medication. As with many illegal drugs, heroin can cause added stress, as a consequence of debt, relationship problems and conflicts with the law (Substance Use and Mental Illness Treatment Team 2009).

Dual diagnosis

Dual diagnosis is a term used to denote the presence of both mental health and substance misuse issues experienced by individuals. It is applied not only to people with severe and complex mental health problems and significant addiction but also to those with mild to moderate mental health problems who may have issues with drugs and/or alcohol, such as a dependent drinker experiencing increasing anxiety or a recreational drug user struggling with low mood after use (DH 2002).

People with combined substance and mental health problems represent a third of mental health service users (Menezes *et al.* 1996) and half of substance use service users (Weaver *et al.* 2001). They often face the problem of being excluded from mental health services because of their substance misuse issues and equally excluded from drug and alcohol services because of their mental health problems.

The substances most used by people with mental health problems are alcohol, cannabis and stimulants. Most are not physically addicted or even dependent on these substances, but their use often exacerbates their mental health issues, which in turn affects their wider issues, such as housing, finances and engagement with services. The complex needs of people with dual diagnosis include their physical health, difficult relationships with families and friends and risk of suicide, violence and victimization (Hughes 2006).

Sexual health

The impact of sex and sexual behaviours on mental health and well-being is wide ranging, from the importance of healthy sexual behaviour in maintaining good emotional health through to the devastating effects of child sexual abuse on an individual's adult mental capacity.

In looking at the evidence for reducing teenage pregnancies for NICE, Trivedi *et al.* (2007) found many studies showing the importance of positive parental relationships, parental involvement in children and positive attitudes to education to be vital in promoting positive sexual health in children and young people. Material circumstances, employment and aspirations for the future also were key elements in developing positive attitudes to self-esteem, decision making and conflict resolution.

A clear relationship between risky sexual behaviour (for example, not using condoms or having several partners) and common psychiatric behaviours has been identified (Kosunen *et al.* 2003; Ramrakha *et al.* 2000). Lehrer *et al.* (2006) found that this was also associated with the use of alcohol and drugs, particularly for females. The link between risky sexual behaviour and low self-esteem is strong, but it is unclear whether low self-esteem results in risky sexual behaviour or is a product of the activity (Ethier *et al.* 2006).

Suicide and self-harm – impact on others

Suicide and self-harm are the focus of Chapter 7. Although only very small numbers of people commit suicide, there are significant direct effects on a very wide group of people, including carers, family and friends, colleagues, and staff in any related services. Among the staff, it is particularly front-line health staff who are affected, although it should be borne in mind that the majority of victims have not been in contact with specialist services. There can also be an impact on someone who finds the victim. If the victim was killed by a train or moving vehicle, the driver could also be seriously affected, a fact long recognized by railway operators and trade unions.

PRINCIPLES INTO PRACTICE

This chapter has focused on the first two of our underlying principles: mental health and well-being is a holistic concept; and it is vital to address the social, economic, political, cultural and environmental factors that enhance mental health and well-being through a consideration of the way these factors impact at different life stages. Each individual has their own genetic predisposition interacting with a complex environment, which produces variation in lifestyle choices. These in turn interact with mental health and well-being. The chapter has also used the third principle of identifying need in specific sections of the population.

Chapter 5

HOW CAN WE DEVELOP MENTAL HEALTH AND WELL-BEING STRATEGICALLY?

KEY POINTS

- Healthy public policy is as important for mental health and well-being as for physical health.
- Strengthening communities is integral to strategic development of mental health and well-being.
- Personal skills development includes:
  - behaviour change
  - 'nudge'
  - social marketing.
- Mental well-being impact assessment is a useful tool for creating supportive environments.
- Strategic reorientation of health services involves:
  - organizational development
  - stepped model of care
  - holistic approaches
  - needs assessment
  - evidence of effectiveness
  - service user and carer involvement
  - integrated care.

INTRODUCTION

As explained in the Introduction, the Ottawa Charter for Health Promotion identified the following five essential areas for action underlying a strategy to fundamentally change health and well-being:

- Build healthy public policy.
- Strengthen community action.
- Develop personal skills.
- Create supportive environments.
- Reorientate services.

(WHO 1986)

These areas for action are discussed in more detail later in this chapter, with a focus on their strategic implications for mental health and well-being. The same areas will be used as headings in Chapter 6, which considers some tools and methods for putting these strategic principles into practice.

One useful tool for strategists when they are reflecting on their approach is to think of two axes: the vertical axis goes from 'authoritative' at the top to 'negotiated' at the bottom; and the horizontal axis goes from 'individual' on the left to 'collective' on the right (Beattie 1991). This creates four sections on to which activities can be mapped. An example of authoritative/individual activity is health persuasion, which contrasts with negotiated/individual activities such as counselling or empowerment. An example of authoritative/collective action is legislative action for health, which contrasts with negotiated/group activity, for example community development in health. This model can be applied to ensure a balance of approaches: if there is a tendency nationally to focus on individual lifestyles such as drinking behaviour, rather than legislative change such as minimum pricing, a strategist may try to address this through local policy on licensing outlets, combined with community-based work. The strategist may also decide to make sure that work addressing individual lifestyle change uses negotiated methods as well as 'top-down' delivery of messages.

BUILD HEALTHY PUBLIC POLICY

Healthy public policy, the first of the Ottawa Charter essential areas for action, means that health is on the agenda of policy makers in all sectors and at all levels, directing them to be aware of the health consequences of their decisions and to accept their responsibilities for health. This may include diverse but complementary approaches, including legislation, fiscal measures, taxation and organizational change. It is coordinated action that leads to health, income and social policies that foster greater equity (WHO 1986).

The move from health service provision for physical illness towards the promotion of physical well-being has a parallel in mental health: it is important to shift attention from mental health service provision to the promotion of mental and emotional health and well-being.

National mental health policies were discussed in Chapter 1. Within our case study chapters we make reference to particular appropriate policies, such as those related to suicide (Chapter 7), children and young people and BME groups (Chapter 8) and long-term conditions (Chapter 9). In this section we consider the wider policy agenda – policy that is not health-specific but can make a huge contribution to improving health (including mental health) and preventing ill health.

Hunter (2003) examined the government's intention to shift the health policy agenda in the UK towards health and away from health care. Among the suggested reasons for failure to achieve this were the need for the involvement of large numbers of different organizations and the need for long-term commitment.

Marmot (2010a) produced six policy objectives to reduce inequalities in health. The first related specifically to children ('Give every child the best start in life' (p.16)), and the second and third to children and working-age adults ('Enable all children, young people and adults to maximize their capabilities and have control over their lives' (p.18) and 'Create fair employment and good work for all' (p.20)). The next two were aimed at the whole community ('Ensure a healthy standard of living for all' (p.22) and 'Create and develop healthy and sustainable places and communities' (p.24)). His final policy objective ('Strengthen the role and impact of ill health prevention' (p.26)) focused on the need for prevention of ill health, rather than on treating illness.

Government fiscal strategy is important for the inequalities agenda. Where government fiscal strategy is to promote the growth of the private sector, there may be ways in which this growth can be channelled to reduce the burden of poverty in cities and regions. Examples include: improving career progression in low-paid, low-skilled retail, catering and care jobs (Devins et al. 2014), local skills strategies (Sissons and Jones

2014) and helping unemployed young people to find private-sector work (Russell, Thompson and Simmons 2014). Such approaches are especially important when families in which at least one adult works have become the largest poverty group in the UK (Schmuecker 2014).

With regard to worklessness issues, as discussed in Chapter 2, Bambra (2011) argues that interventions at the macro level are likely to be more effective than interventions that mitigate harm at an organizational or individual level. For example, the recommendation to implement a Minimum Income for Healthy Living (Marmot 2010b) would be such an intervention. Bambra also suggests that interventions designed to increase levels of work among those with long-term conditions may be effective if they include workplace design or working hours, as well as addressing individual skills in job search and application. Establishing a living wage and addressing the health-related aspects of worklessness are chosen as two out of nine top-priority actions to tackle inequalities in a collection entitled *If You Could do One Thing* (British Association for the Humanities and Social Sciences 2014).

In England, as mentioned in the Introduction, health policy transferred leadership for health and well-being to the Local Authorities from April 2013. At the same time, since 2009 the government has set out an austerity programme to tackle the recession and the budget deficit through reduced Local Authority budgets, and welfare reform to set up a unified system, and to reduce benefits paid. In the foreword to an assessment of the impact of the economic downturn and policy changes on health inequalities in London, Sir Michael Marmot says:

> Improving health and reducing health inequalities in this macro-economic environment is going to be a great challenge. Rising unemployment, poorer working conditions, depressed incomes and an inability to pay for decent housing and basic needs will all increase negative mental and physical health outcomes across the social gradient and especially for more vulnerable groups. (UCL Institute of Health Equity 2012, p.3)

Stuckler and Basu (2013) use international comparisons to show that the austerity approach costs thousands of lives. They develop the argument that proper consideration of the impacts of austerity, compared with a stimulus approach to managing recession, includes health and not only economic growth. They describe the way Active

Labour Market Programmes (ALMPs) have been shown to protect mental health during recession: in Finland in 2002, among people who had lost their jobs, those who received help from a skilled case-worker providing support, skills and practical help to develop a return to work plan were significantly less likely to show symptoms of depression and anxiety than those who simply received written information. The authors have made comparisons across Europe and found that ALMPs are consistently linked with protection against suicide rates across all European countries, in a way that other social programmes (e.g. health care services, childcare support, housing subsidies, old-age pensions) are not.

Policy concerned with equity and equality is also highly relevant to mental well-being: stigma and discrimination have been mentioned as causes of stress and mental ill health. Much policy and guidance now makes explicit reference to equity and equality, including the Equality Act 2010's 'protected characteristics' (age, disability, gender reassignment, marriage and civil partnership, pregnancy and maternity, race, religion and belief, sex and sexual orientation). For example, most NICE guidelines stress that stigma and discrimination must be avoided and that staff need to be respectful of and sensitive to service users' gender, sexual orientation, socio-economic status, age, background (including cultural, ethnic and religious background) and any disability (NCCMH 2012a).

We hope that it becomes evident throughout this book that policy designed primarily to address problems in topic areas such as housing, employment, children's issues, education, crime, equality and the environment can also have far-reaching effects on mental health and well-being.

STRENGTHEN COMMUNITY ACTION

Concrete and effective community action in setting priorities, making decisions, planning strategies and implementing them to achieve better health is the second area for action of the Ottawa Charter. At the heart of this process is the ownership and control of communities' own endeavours and destinies (WHO 1986).

Communities

In thinking about this aspect of strategy and its application to mental health and well-being, it is useful first to say what we mean by 'community'. Traditionally we think of a community as the people living in a particular geographical area. However, communities may define themselves in many different ways. *The Penguin English Dictionary* (Allen 1986) gives several definitions:

- a group of people living in a particular area
- all the interacting populations of various living organisms in a particular area
- a group of individuals with some common characteristic, for example profession, religion or status
- a body of people or nations having a common history or common interests.

People can be members of several communities. It is important to recognize that communities should not be externally identified for people. People must be able to choose which communities they identify with. A useful categorization of communities recognized by health authorities is as follows:

- the general public
- service users, such as GP patients and mental health service users
- geographical localities, such as neighbourhoods and villages
- communities of interest, such as BME groups and carers.

(Based on Smithies and Webster 1998)

Local communities are not homogeneous entities, but are dynamic and ever changing. They are made up of multiple groups, with interrelated differences, including gender, age, religion, ethnicity, wealth and power. There may also be conflicting local interests. Often projects identify local leaders, but these may not be representative of the rest of the local population: those who are most articulate are rarely those in greatest need. Jewkes and Murcott (1998) found that the 'community' was frequently represented by voluntary sector organizations, which are often made up of professionals, not people from the community they profess to represent.

Strengthening community actions involves addressing issues from the community's viewpoint, which relies on an understanding of the many factors that affect it, including:

- physical aspects: number and location of the people involved and where they can meet (even if it is not a geographical community)
- infrastructure: transport systems, access to communication systems such as broadband and telephone
- patterns of settlement: locations of houses, shops, workplaces
- demographics of the community: age, gender, race and ethnicity, marital status, education, disability, sexual orientation, numbers in households, etc.
- history: established or recently formed community, conflicts and factions within it.

(Based on Hampton and Heaven 2013)

Working from a local perspective entails making sure that the community is engaged, whether it is geographically located or based on a mutual interest. Gaining a general idea of the community's strengths and assets ensures that the starting point is positive, rather than beginning with the gaps and deficiencies.

Understanding and describing communities is the starting point for community development work, which supports the development of strong communities that can identify and use their assets to improve the quality of community life and promote social justice (Scottish Community Development Centre for Learning Connections 2007).

Community development

Empowerment is considered a key aspect of a more holistic view of health and is generally considered to be the process by which a person gains control of his or her life (Rissell 1994). Community development is an approach that seeks to empower individuals, by identifying and developing the skills people need to effect change in their lives. Such skills are often focused on building political power through the formation of social groups working for a common outcome (Scottish Community Development Centre 2011). It is essentially a 'bottom-up' approach, starting with the needs of the community, as identified by them, rather than 'top-down', where 'experts' or politicians make decisions about what is best for a community. The actual activity of empowering a community in itself promotes emotional and mental well-being (Glasgow Centre for Population Health 2011).

This approach is concerned with action that helps people understand and develop their ability to organize themselves in order to respond to issues that they identify as being of importance to them:

> Community development is about building active and sustainable communities based on social justice and mutual respect. It is about changing power structures to remove the barriers that prevent people from participating in the issues that affect their lives. Community workers support individuals, groups and organisations in this process. (SCCD 2001, p.5)

Community development seeks to engage all parts of the community and address barriers to participation, particularly for those most vulnerable and excluded. This involves ensuring that all voices are heard, not just the voices of the most dominant and confident. It is a process that needs time and commitment: it is ongoing, not a short-term answer to problems. It recognizes the interconnectedness of communities and that a holistic approach is crucial. Key values core to the community development process include social justice, self-determination and working and learning together (Community Development Cymru 2007).

The Standing Conference for Community Development (SCCD 2001) identifies several commitments for action, which include: challenging inequalities, power imbalances and discrimination within organizations, communities and in the wider society; ensuring working practice and policy is environmentally sound; encouraging networking between individuals, communities and organizations, and promoting access and choice for all; working from the perspectives of communities and influencing policies affecting those communities; and supporting collective action.

In Chapter 6 we will look at different methods that have been developed to take these principles into practice, including asset-based community development, social capital and social networks. The empowerment that is fundamental to a community development approach is central to mental health and well-being.

DEVELOP PERSONAL SKILLS

The third of the Ottawa Charter areas for action is to develop personal skills. Supporting personal and social development through providing information, education for health and enhancing life skills increases the options available to people to exercise more control over their own health and over their environments, and to make choices conducive to health (WHO 1986).

The relationship between community development and building personal skills is a close one: people within a community develop skills both individually and collectively. In this section we will touch briefly on what is known about behaviour change.

Model of behaviour change

As discussed in Chapter 4, there are links between mental health and well-being and health-related behaviours: smoking, drinking, healthy eating, being physically active, drug-taking and sexual health. Finding ways of changing some of these behaviours is therefore likely to have a positive effect on mental well-being.

Prochaska and DiClemente published their influential Transtheoretical Model of behaviour change in 1984 and a further study was produced ten years later (Prochaska *et al.* 1994), applying the decision-making process to 12 problem behaviours. The model has become fundamental to the delivery of health improvement services in the UK. The 'stages of change' involved in adopting a new behaviour can be described as:

- pre-contemplation (not ready to change)
- contemplation (thinking of change)
- preparation (ready to change)
- action (making change)
- maintenance (staying on track)
- relapse (fall from grace).

(Nursing Theories 2012)

The stages are relevant to both the individual and a helper. The model's strength is in identifying pre-contemplation and contemplation stages in advance of preparation for and ultimately making a decision to change behaviour. Planning for and maintaining the change form an important part of the support a 'helper' can offer, using theory about environmental prompts, the importance of establishing rewards and asking for allies. The model also means a 'helper' does not try to rush to behaviour change where someone is in the pre-contemplation stage.

There are also courses that develop personal skills to improve mental health directly, such as: assertiveness, coping with depression and dealing with stress (see Chapter 6).

'Nudge'

A nudge is:

> Any aspect of the choice architecture that alters people's behaviour in a predictable way without forbidding any options or significantly changing their economic incentives. To count as a mere nudge, the intervention must be easy and cheap to avoid. Nudges are not mandates. Putting the fruit at eye level counts as a nudge. Banning junk food does not. (Thaler and Sunstein 2008, reprinted 2009, p.6)

This is similar to the 'action' stage of the behaviour change model quoted above, where the person is seeking the prompts for the behaviour they want to change, and deciding to avoid them. The theory of 'nudge' is based on six design principles of good choice architecture, which can be applied to many aspects of human behaviour:

> INcentives: benefits now; for example, watching the 'calories burned' meter

> Understand mappings: link a choice to its effect; for example, the fly in the urinal in the airport at Schiphol in Amsterdam improved aim by 80 per cent

> Defaults: the 'do nothing' option is the line of least resistance; for example, automatic subscription updates to gyms

> Give feedback: tell people when they are making mistakes; for example, medication that makes recovering alcoholics sick when they imbibe alcohol

> Expect error: humans make mistakes, so design to allow for them; for example, 'look right' warning signs at pedestrian crossings

Structure complex choices: for example, suggest changes based on similar choices already made; if you can give up cigarettes you can exercise more, too. (Adapted from Thaler and Sunstein 2008, reprinted 2009, p.109)

Applying the principles of good design to encourage desired behaviour is a useful concept as one component of a strategy, and may be seen as a link between personal skills and the fourth action area of 'creating supportive environments', discussed in the next section. Before that, we finish this section on personal skills development with a brief look at social marketing.

Social marketing

In recent years, the importance of social marketing as a strategic tool has also developed.

Social marketing is the systematic application of commercial marketing tools to the design, implementation and evaluation of health and social behaviour change programmes. Health-related social marketing is 'the systematic application of marketing concepts and techniques, to achieve specific behavioural goals to improve health and reduce health inequalities' (National Consumer Council and National Social Marketing Centre 2006, p.39).

Social marketing focuses on target groups within the population, tailoring campaigns and awareness, based on consumer research and insight (French, Blair-Stevens and McVey 2010). It aims to tackle inequalities by reaching groups of the population not easily influenced or motivated by other means, and enabling communication with them on their own terms.

Social marketing includes mapping client populations, often using the same 'segments' as defined for commercial marketing purposes. This may stimulate health and other professionals to focus clearly on a specific target group and consider cultural issues such as their aspirations, or the media they are most likely to use.

Social marketing might be particularly helpful in relation to moving people from pre-contemplation to contemplation of change in the model above, and sometimes in actually making the change.

In terms of personal skills development it is important to appreciate the role and limitations of behaviour change models and social marketing, both of which assume that the selected behaviour change is the principal measure of success. This contrasts with the community capacity building approach, where the development of skills and networks is seen as the main goal, with the possibility of choosing healthier lifestyles as a consequence of increased confidence and self-belief.

CREATE SUPPORTIVE ENVIRONMENTS

The fourth of the Ottawa Charter areas for action is creating supportive environments. Health cannot be separated from other goals in our complex and interrelated societies. Patterns of life, work and leisure should be developed to create conditions that are safe, stimulating, satisfying and enjoyable (WHO 1986).

This requires a consideration of the effect on human development at the time when decisions are made about resources, policies, plans, programmes, workforce, land use, and transport systems. How do we create an environment that enhances health and well-being? This section will consider briefly the role Health Impact Assessment (HIA) may play in this process, with a focus on mental health and well-being.

Health Impact Assessment and well-being

There are several different types of Impact Assessment (IA): health IA, economic IA, environmental IA, social IA, sustainability IA, risk assessment and integrated IA. A review of these methods (Brown, Shassere and Sengupta 2005) found that because the techniques are analytical, they tend to be relatively straightforward to use. Simple, step-by-step processes can be developed. This adds to the ease of carrying out any policy assessment, possibly allowing a wider range of people to be involved than more complex processes. In addition, the assessments potentially increase the bank of evidence available for subsequent policy development.

We are focusing in this subsection on HIA. A wide variety of tools has been developed for practitioners to use (HIA Gateway 2013). Most of these include some way of identifying distributed impact within the population and in this way link up with equality and diversity issues. This is important because of the legal requirement in the UK (under the Equality Act 2010) to assess the impact of policies and services on minority groups. Coordinating activity in this area with HIA at a population level is important. Evidence is still being developed about the effectiveness of HIA as an approach (Harris-Roxas *et al.* 2012).

Some of the available tools, but not all, pay particular attention to the mental health and well-being aspects as part of the assessment. HIA is more effective than either sustainability appraisal or environmental appraisal at ensuring that mental health and well-being are addressed in spatial plans (Gray *et al.* 2011).

As mentioned in the Introduction, England's Health and Social Care Act 2012 has given local authorities a new responsibility for health and well-being. The new role entails 'including health in all policies so that each decision seeks the most health benefit for the investment' and encouraging 'health promoting environments, for example access to green spaces and transport' (DH 2011c, p.3).

The NHS Confederation (2012) has recognized the potential for HIA as a useful approach for the Health and Wellbeing Boards, the statutory body created to help fulfil this responsibility. This may raise the profile of HIA as a tool to demonstrate systematic assessment of the impact of decisions about resources, spatial planning and policies on health and well-being in England.

A case study from Gateshead recognized that embedding HIA into strategic corporate thinking requires high-level support, using the existing local infrastructure and linking HIA to the local strategic vision for the area (Learmonth and Curtis 2012).

Mental Wellbeing Impact Assessment and resilience

Interest in improving mental well-being through IA has been growing over the last ten years. A report from WHO Europe working with the Mental Health Foundation recommends that every policy should be scrutinized for its impact on mental health and well-being. This is one way to begin to address the strong two-way relationship between poor mental health and a range of social, educational and economic problems (Friedli 2009). A recent publication that builds on this development work is the *Mental Wellbeing Impact Assessment: A Toolkit for Wellbeing* (Cooke *et al.* 2011). The toolkit is an excellent resource to help address the strong links between inequalities and mental health identified in

Chapter 2. This work is closely linked with the field of resilience theory, which has developed rapidly over the last ten years to explain why some communities and individuals prevail despite adversity, and to explore whether interventions to teach or develop resilience are effective. One definition of resilience identifies three elements: resistance (sustained adaptive effort despite challenge), recovery (bouncing back from a challenge) and re-bound (growth and learning to expand knowledge and skills) (Kent, Davis and Reich 2014).

At a community level:

Resilience reflects the extent to which communities are able to exercise informal social controls or come together to tackle common problems. It is people's social networks, more than any physical characteristics of place, that appear to be most crucial in creating a sense of attachment to place. (Taylor 2008, p.7)

The Mental Wellbeing Impact Assessment (MWIA) Toolkit draws from the developing literature about resilience for individuals and communities. The framework for assessing the impact on mental health is based on:

- enhancing control (including finance, the living environment and ability to influence external decisions)
- reducing anxiety (including communication, integrated services and informal support)
- facilitating participation and promoting inclusion (having a valued role, a sense of belonging, tackling stigma and discrimination, and social networks).

A linked report (Cooke and Stansfield 2009) gives a number of examples of the impact that MWIA has had. The outcomes from undertaking MWIA have been positive and suggest that MWIA has an important role to play in improving well-being through: more responsive services; shared understanding of well-being among partners; activities all being scrutinized to maximize the ways they improve mental well-being; engaging stakeholders in the co-production of well-being; and involving communities in assessing need and identifying suitable indicators for improvement.

REORIENTATE SERVICES

The fifth of the Ottawa Charter areas for action is the challenge of reorientating health and social care services to create a system that contributes to the pursuit of health. This responsibility is shared among individuals, community groups, health professionals, health service institutions and governments. The health sector must move beyond clinical and curative services to support the needs of individuals and communities for a healthier life, and open channels with the broader social, political, economic and physical environmental components (WHO 1986). This continues to apply to mental health services as well as other aspects of health care.

In 2002 Derek Wanless, former chair of the Westminster Bank, was asked to carry out a review for the Chancellor of the technological, demographic and medical trends over the following 20 years in the UK likely to impact on health service provision, and identify financial and other resources required for the NHS to provide a publicly funded high-quality service (Wanless 2002). The review recognized the economic imperative to change the way the health service operated. It stressed the need for effective use of resources and the importance in this context of disease prevention.

From a technical public health perspective there are key tools to help with service reorientation: effective health care needs assessment at a population level to inform strategic service planning; and the application of evidence about effectiveness to inform the choice of intervention. Both of these tools are applied in a political context, and skills in relationship building and brokering are essential. Maintaining a close connection with user feedback and quality measures is the final tool essential for service change. A strategic approach will have these three building blocks beneath it, brought together through an organizational development process, using quality markers and user feedback to ensure that progress on the ground is meaningful. While these tools are not sufficient to achieve transformational change, they underpin development of cost-effective services to improve health.

After outlining the principles of organizational development, this section describes the stepped-care model for mental health and the recovery model, and then discusses the two tools of health care needs assessment and applying evidence about what works at a policy level. Finally it touches on the role of user feedback and quality assurance in terms of a strategy for change.

Organizational development

A key part of reorientating health services is organizational development, starting with the leaders in the whole system, and working to focus and drive change at all levels of the organization and with its partners. England's Health Inequalities National Support Team, as part of their work on systematic improvement of organizational behaviour, identified ten major lessons from their work:

- make vision and strategy clear
- strengthen primary care use
- extend leadership and engagement
- make partnership work
- get system and scale right
- adjust workforce
- be proactive in seeking out the thousands of people who already have disease or are at high risk but are accessing services sub-optimally or not at all
- capitalize on community engagement
- reduce variation in performance, by raising the performance of the lower achievers
- use population health intelligence.

(Adapted from Bentley 2008)

Stepped model of care

The stepped-care model has two principles, based on NICE guidance. The first is a good chance of expected positive outcomes, balanced with a minimal level of inconvenience or hardship to the patient. The second is regular review, with a variety of possible actions: continuing with the existing treatment, transfer or 'stepping up' to more intensive treatments, 'stepping down' to less intensive treatment, 'stepping out' to an alternative form of treatment, or no treatment (IAPT n.d.).

The stepped model of care is one of the ways organizational change theory has been applied to mental health services. It entails starting at the first-line treatment and moving onto more complex treatment if the former is not effective – that is, stepping care up (or down) the pathway in accordance with the needs of the client and their response to the treatment. NICE (2011a) recommends the use of a stepped-care model to provide the most effective services for people with common mental health problems. More intensive or extensive forms of therapy may be essential for some people with complex issues.

Holistic approaches: the recovery model

In mental health, the term 'recovery' has a slightly different interpretation from that applied to physical health. It is more about people staying in control of their lives in spite of having mental health problems, and this is commonly known as the recovery model. 'The recovery model aims to help people with mental health problems to look beyond mere survival and existence. It encourages them to move forward, set new goals and do things and develop relationships that give their lives meaning' (Mental Health Foundation n.d. c).

This positive thinking is linked to a holistic approach, not only addressing the mental health condition but looking at other aspects of life, as discussed in Chapters 2, 3 and 4. Progress may be measured by use of a recovery star, as outlined in Chapter 1.

Needs assessment

The aim of health care needs assessment is to provide information to plan, negotiate and change services for the better and improve health in other ways. A working definition of 'health care need' is 'the population's ability to benefit from health care' (Stevens *et al.* 2004, p.6). Each element of the definition is important:

- The population's ability to benefit from health care is the sum total of individuals' ability to benefit.

- The ability to benefit does not mean every outcome is guaranteed to be favourable, but on average the intervention is effective.

- The benefit is not just clinical status but can include social factors such as reassurance, or supportive care.

- Health care includes all stages of treatment, including prevention, addressing diagnosis, continuing care, rehabilitation and possibly palliative care.

(Adapted from Stevens *et al.* 2004)

This process involves:

- assessment of incidence and prevalence (how many people need the service or intervention?)
- assessment of effectiveness and cost-effectiveness of the services (do they confer any benefit and, if so, at what cost?)
- assessment of baseline services (which existing services need to change and what are the opportunities and resources to make change happen?).

(Adapted from Stevens *et al.* 2004)

It is a core part of this process that evidence of effectiveness of the interventions is considered. We will describe further in the next subsection how the two processes (needs assessment and drawing on the evidence) interlock.

As mentioned in the Introduction, in England there is a statutory requirement to produce Joint Strategic Needs Assessments (JSNAs) to examine what the local community needs in terms of health care and social care, and a Joint Strategy Health and Wellbeing (JHWS). This has led to a variety of approaches in different areas of England, albeit with many common elements. They consider the wide range of factors that have an impact on the population's health and well-being, for example those factors discussed in Chapters 2 and 3. The JSNA draws together at a local level the sorts of issues that would be expected from Chapters 2, 3 and 4, with some of the information sources and outcomes from Chapter 1. It also applies evidence of effectiveness, which is discussed in the next subsection.

With the range of intelligence presented in a JSNA, or more specific needs assessments in other parts of the UK, decision-makers can begin to identify priorities. This is likely to be a political process, in which local knowledge and understanding also play a large part. The NHS Confederation has identified ten key questions for Health and Wellbeing Boards to ask themselves about their JHWS, starting with: is the JHWS being co-created through active engagement and involvement of local communities, patients, service users and carers? Two key questions in terms of this book follow later: is the JHWS sufficiently ambitious in addressing well-being and not just health? and is a system approach being taken to align resources with strategic priorities? (NHS Confederation 2013).

An Internet search suggests there is variety in JHWS developed since the requirement to produce them came into force in April 2013. Systematic scrutiny of their scope, scale and success over the next few years will be a fruitful area for further research.

Evidence of effectiveness

The second public health lever for change is consistently using evidence of effectiveness. The National Institute for Health and Care Excellence (NICE; formerly National Institute for Health and Clinical Excellence) has the role of providing guidance on evidence in England, and the Knowledge Network is the equivalent in Scotland. In some places, we have used single research studies (reliably scrutinized, that is, in peer-reviewed journals), but where possible systematic reviews[5] or meta-analyses[6] have been used to inform the statements in Chapters 2 and 3, and the three extended case study chapters.

NICE describes the process it has developed for systematically reviewing 'the best available scientific evidence':

> The randomised controlled trial (RCT) is normally the most appropriate source of evidence for judging the 'efficacy' of clearly circumscribed interventions that are implemented in ideal circumstances. However, such evidence is not always available or appropriate: it might not be feasible to conduct RCTs for some complex, large-scale, multi-agency and multi-faceted interventions, policies and services; and in some cases it may be unethical to do so. Further, given the complexity of causal chains in public health, the external validity of some RCT findings often has to be enhanced by observational studies to determine the 'effectiveness' of interventions in real-life situations. For evaluating large-scale interventions, observational studies may be the only feasible option. (NICE 2012a)

---

5   A systematic review is the critical assessment and evaluation of research that attempts to address a focused question using methods designed to reduce the likelihood of bias. 'Whenever a systematic review is conducted, explicit methods are used to locate primary studies, and explicit criteria are used to assess their quality' (Aceijas 2011, p.25).

6   '[A] meta analysis will thoroughly examine a number of valid studies on a topic and combine the results using accepted statistical methodology as if they were from one large study' (Aceijas 2011, p.25).

The Medical Research Council (MRC) has produced guidance on evaluating complex interventions (Craig *et al.* 2008) and using natural experiments to evaluate population health interventions (Craig *et al.* 2011).

In public health, qualitative social scientific evidence, as well as clinical and epidemiological evidence, is used to examine outcomes, context, process and implementation (along with barriers to and facilitators for interventions). There is little academic consensus about how best to synthesize these different approaches and there is still less agreement about how to use these disciplines to develop guidance. NICE has developed a process involving stakeholders at critical stages of the process of sifting and synthesizing the evidence.

Increasingly, work is going on to ensure that research-based knowledge about effectiveness and cost effectiveness is actually used in practice. Different infrastructure is being developed internationally to support policy-makers, organizations and practitioners in making best use of systematically reviewed evidence (Armstrong *et al.* 2013; LaRocca *et al.* 2013).

Public health professionals are expected to be able to demonstrate their competence in skills of sourcing evidence, critical appraisal and assessing cost-effectiveness analysis (Aceijas 2011). However, in practice, the first step should always be to see what systematically reviewed appraisals already exist, because their findings will be more robust than a local 'quick and dirty' assessment.

In England, the use of commissioning provides one way to try to make this work at a system level, rather than with individual practitioners or groups of practitioners. This 'scaling up' of what we know works is an important part of tackling inequalities. The approach has relevance to decision-makers in other parts of the UK working at a strategic level, albeit with different planning tools and processes.

A flow chart for evidence-based decision making is shown in Figure 5.1. It developed over a number of years in Gateshead as a means to create system change through including evidence at the development stage of the commissioning process. Where evidence is strong it should be included in specifications, monitoring and quality assurance requirements, and where evidence is weak, resources for evaluation should be included in the contract. A number of principles essential for this work were identified, including:

- proactive engagement with all stakeholders
- building quality standards based on accredited evidence into service specifications
- including views of patients, carers and service users
- supporting realignment or decommissioning of ineffective services
- building capacity of key stakeholders including providers as part of ongoing organizational development.

(Learmonth 2013)

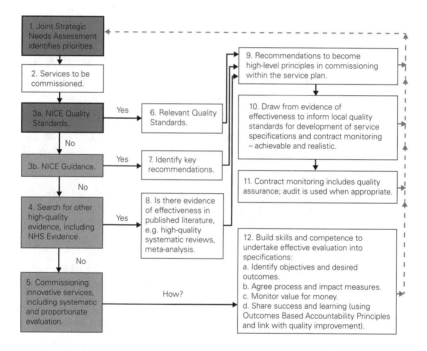

Figure 5.1: Flow chart for evidence-based commissioning

One of the major advantages of this model, in addition to its ability to 'scale up' evidence-based interventions, is that it provides a clear decision point about the resource required to enable implementation to be realistically carried out and appropriately monitored. If the intervention being commissioned is not evidence based, it provides the same clarity about evaluation at the start of the process. This, in turn, should help generate rigorous evaluation, to feed into future research agendas. WHO recommended that a figure of 10 per cent of an investment in innovative services be identified for evaluation purposes (WHO Regional Office for Europe 1998). The evaluation process is discussed in Chapter 6.

In places where commissioning is not the chosen method of strategic service planning, this early application of evidence, working with service providers, should still be useful at an appropriate stage.

If there is a strong evidence base then there should be a quality assurance system in the organization to ensure that the recommended process is being correctly implemented, or that the recommended service is being adequately delivered to be effective. Key elements of such a system are the following:

- 'Audit' – an examination or review that establishes the extent to which a condition, process or performance conforms to predetermined standards or criteria. Audits can be particularly useful in assessing certain aspects of mental health. They make use of suitably qualified experts who consider a range of information or evidence to assess a service or a process. Health Equity Audits are discussed in Chapter 6. A particularly relevant audit for mental health is a Suicide Audit. Given that suicide reduction is a key element of mental health strategy, even though there are only small numbers, it is important to gain as much knowledge as possible about the 'how', the 'why', the 'where', the 'who', the 'what' and the 'when' of suicide cases. Suicide audits are discussed in Chapter 7.

- 'Quality' – the level of performance that characterizes the service provided. Ultimately measures of quality are based upon value judgements, but there are ingredients and determinants of quality that can be measured objectively. These ingredients and determinants have been classified by Donabedian (1969) into measures of structure such as manpower and facilities; processes such as diagnostic and therapeutic procedures; and outcomes such as case fatality rates, disability rates and user satisfaction. The last of these – user satisfaction – is particularly crucial in relation to mental health, as discussed in the next subsection.

- 'Quality assurance' – the system of procedures, checks, audits and corrective actions in place. Quality control is the supervision and control of all operations in a process to detect and correct systematic or excessively random variations.

(Adapted from Last 1995, p.11 and p.136)

All Mental Health Trusts in England have to work towards objectives defined by the current No Health without Mental Health Strategy (HM Government and DH 2011) discussed in Chapter 1. There is currently considerable attention being paid to 'Payment by Results', to try to encourage more focus on outcomes. At the same time, the National Institute for Health and Care Excellence is producing Quality Standards based on evidence on a wide variety of subjects, including, for example, alcohol, drug use and anxiety disorders.

Service user and carer involvement

Fundamental to the reorientation of health services is systematic use of the views of users and carers. This is one of the most important ways in which high-quality services can be developed through listening to the user's voice; at the same time, being heard, in itself, enhances self-esteem.

Since Community Health Councils were established in 1973, the notion of user involvement has become established in NHS policy. The NHS and Community Care Act was the first legislation to require user involvement in service planning in 1990, and subsequent policies, such as the Patient's Charter and Local Voices, have stressed the importance of services involving patients and responding to their needs (Tait and Lester 2005).

Mental health policies now tend to stress the need for patient and user involvement; for example, Wales's mental health strategy (Welsh Government 2012, p.27) refers to 'a new partnership with the public', with desired outcomes of: equitable access for vulnerable groups with those protected characteristics; access to linguistically appropriate treatment for Welsh speakers; reduced stigma and discrimination; and greater (and effective) public engagement in the planning, delivery and evaluation of local mental health services.

NICE guidance (NCCMH 2012a) suggests key requirements for high-quality service user experience, including:

- involvement in decisions and respect for preferences
- clear, comprehensible information and support for self-care
- emotional support, empathy and respect
- fast access to reliable health advice

- effective treatment delivered by trained professionals
- attention to physical and environmental needs
- involvement of, and support for, family and carers
- continuity of care and smooth transitions.

User or carer involvement in services is often considered intrinsically useful, but most people consider the value of such an approach to lie in the difference it can make to the individuals, or the service. Benefits may be in terms of the individual, such as increasing their social networks or empowering them, or of the service, such as improving relationships between users and carers and staff, making services more appropriate or responsive (Simpson and House 2003).

There is a wide range of ways that users and carers may be involved, from individuals telling their stories, via websites such as Patients Opinion or through developing person-centred approaches to care (Cook and Miller 2012), to full involvement in research (Repper, Simpson and Grimshaw 2011) and developing training materials (Repper and Breeze 2006). We discuss the 'how' further in Chapter 6.

Integrated care

Mental health policies increasingly stress the need for services to be integrated, so that patients are on a clear pathway of care, without unnecessary or difficult transitions between services. For example, Northern Ireland's standard 19 (DHSS&PS 2011) says:

> A person using mental health services should have an integrated care pathway for their assessment, treatment, care and ongoing management where health and social care (including primary care) work in partnership with users and their carers to develop the most appropriate and accessible services. (p.16)

Wales's strategy (Welsh Government 2012) describes a fully integrated network of care, such that service users experience a more integrated approach from those delivering services. The benefits of integrated care are many. For the patient, it is much easier and more comfortable if movement between settings or agencies flows smoothly, with all agencies understanding the situation and reducing the need for the patient to repeat the same story time and again or to have to make their own arrangements to move to the next stage. For the services involved, a clearer picture of the whole situation helps in assessing the patient's needs and future pathway. Integrated working also reduces the amount of duplication of services that can sometimes be seen, and can clarify the roles of each organization.

PRINCIPLES INTO PRACTICE

In this chapter we have focused on the strategic application of our four key principles. The chapter is based on our broad definition of mental health, and the need to include social, economic, cultural and environmental determinants of health, for example through mental health and well-being impact assessment. The chapter touches on the relationship between mental health and well-being and other aspects of health-related behaviour, particularly in the section on personal skills. The chapter goes on to provide the theoretical underpinning for principles three and four, discussing the way in which assessment of need, systematically reviewed evidence of effectiveness and user involvement give invaluable help in re-shaping priorities for mental health and well-being.

In conclusion, this chapter has set out some strategic considerations in relation to mental health and well-being, using a framework that encompasses healthy public policy, strengthening communities, changing personal behaviours, creating supportive environments and reorientating services. The goal has been to establish the 'why'. The next chapter will pick up each of these strands of activity and identify the 'what' and the 'how'.

Chapter 6

HOW CAN WE DEVELOP MENTAL HEALTH AND WELL-BEING OPERATIONALLY?

KEY POINTS

This chapter identifies effective interventions for the at-risk groups described in Chapter 3.

- Implementation of a strategy for mental health and well-being requires strong programmes of capacity building in both communities and organizations.

- Building on assets is a contested concept but lies within the community development tradition; it is not a replacement for services.

- Strengthening communities may also draw on understanding of social capital, social networks and co-production.

- Developing personal skills includes a range of training programmes to enhance self-esteem and self-confidence, positive mental health and happiness networks, health literacy and continuing education as well as lifestyle-specific activity.

- Creating supportive environments involves working in settings and enhancing the skills of the people who work in them.

- Examples of reorientating health services include social prescribing, dealing with depression, and service user and carer involvement.

- Health Equity Audit is an important tool to ensure services are targeted to those who need them most.

- Evaluation is an important tool for building evidence for innovative or hard-to-measure services.

INTRODUCTION

This chapter takes each of the five areas for action for strategic planning discussed in Chapter 5 and re-visits them in terms of the practical implications for organizations and practitioners in terms of the methods and approaches that may be used in service delivery. The headings in this chapter match those in Chapter 5:

- build healthy public policy
- strengthen community action
- develop personal skills
- create supportive environments
- reorientate Health Services.

(WHO 1986)

Effective interventions related to the at-risk groups described in Chapter 3 are identified under 'create supportive environments'. We have largely excluded the wide range of effective services that come under health care because treatment is not the main focus of this book.

BUILD HEALTHY PUBLIC POLICY

Healthy public policy, as the name suggests, is mainly concerned with national and local policy decisions, such as discussed in Chapter 5. Policy may impact very directly on service configuration: across the UK, there are policy drivers to ensure that integration of services becomes a reality. For example, the Public Bodies (Joint Working) (Scotland) Bill 2013 'provides the framework which will support the improvement of the quality and consistency of health and social care services in Scotland' (Scottish Parliamentary Corporate Body 2013, p.2). This will be done through:

- nationally agreed outcomes, focusing on older people
- joint accountability across health and social care
- integrated budgets
- local service planning groups. (The Scottish Government 2013)

The establishment in England of Health and Wellbeing Boards with their statutory responsibilities described in the Introduction may also be considered part of healthy public policy.

Organizations can influence the development of healthy public policy. Lobbying to improve policy at this level may be seen by some groups as an important part of their role, particularly voluntary sector groups lobbying on single issues such as tobacco or food. Organizations and practitioners tend to work within the constraints set by policy-makers, so it can be beneficial to them to change the direction of policy.

STRENGTHEN COMMUNITY ACTION

In Chapter 5 we discussed this, the second of the Ottawa Charter areas for action, in terms of the nature of communities, the principles underlying community development, and the way these can be taken forward through community capacity building. In this section we look at some ways that the principles of community development have been developed in terms of practical approaches:

- building on assets, including participatory appraisal, appreciative inquiry and asset mapping
- social capital
- social networks
- co-production
- capacity building.

Building on assets

There is increasing evidence that using an asset-based approach can enhance the quality of information that is collected, by focusing on local people's perceptions, and can improve the services that are subsequently provided, by basing them on what people want. It has been described as 'a glass half-full' approach (Foot with Hopkins 2010).

An asset-based approach starts with people's energy, skills, interests, knowledge and life experience (Glasgow Centre for Population Health 2011). It aims to enable people to rely less on public services by empowering them (Sigerson and Gruer 2011). People are not seen as passive recipients of services, but as active citizens, who have a range of assets that can be drawn on to improve health and health services.

Assets have been described at three levels:

- Individual level: resilience, self-esteem and sense of purpose, commitment to learning.
- Community level: family and friendship or supportive networks, intergenerational solidarity, community cohesion, religious tolerance and harmony.
- Organizational level: environmental resources necessary for promoting physical, mental and social health, employment security and opportunity for voluntary service, religious tolerance and harmony, safe and pleasant housing, political democracy and social justice.

(Based on Morgan and Ziglio 2007)

Engagement is a key element of developing an asset-based approach. Effective involvement can improve provision, reduce unnecessary medical consultations and make the best use of limited services. It helps to ensure that services are responsive to need and are accessible and acceptable, thereby reducing non-attendance and subsequent costs. Involving people in decisions about their own health can boost self-confidence and self-efficacy, as well as improve decision making. The engagement approach is based on the principles of community development described in Chapter 5.

Critics argue that the approach may distract from fundamental questions of power and access to resources:

> If the strength of the assets movement is that it has generated discussion about redressing the balance of power between the public sector, public services and local communities, its fatal weakness has been the failure to question the balance of power between public services, communities and corporate interests. As such, asset-based approaches sound the drum beat for the retreat of statutory, state provision of both public services and public health. (Friedli 2012, p.10)

We acknowledge that this view may be a useful counter to the idea that community-based assets replace services. However, community development is from a radical tradition, and we consider that asset building may be developed in the appropriate way within that tradition, rather than being a way in which the state can opt out of service provision.

Participatory appraisal, appreciative inquiry and asset mapping are all techniques used in asset-based community development, and are also used to explore the strengths within communities from an asset-based perspective.

Participatory appraisal is based on the principles of empowerment and ownership of the development process. It seeks to improve the world by understanding it and then changing it, by the collective reflective inquiry of participants. Actions that flow from this reflection will be influenced by culture, local context and social relationships. A key feature is that local people are trained to research the knowledge, views and experience within their neighbourhood, which leads to them having increased control over their lives (Baum, MacDougall and Smith 2006).

Appreciative inquiry is a method of asking questions that focus on strengths and what is done well, rather than on what is done badly. It is based on the idea that an organization that makes inquiries into problems will continue to find problems but, in contrast, one that explores and appreciates what is best within it will find more of what is good, providing a sound basis on which to build a new future (Seel 2008).

The main differences between appreciative inquiry and the usual approach of focusing on problems are the following:

- Problem solving identifies felt need, while appreciative inquiry appreciates what is currently the best.
- Problem solving identifies and analyses causes, while appreciative inquiry imagines the possible future.
- Problem solving identifies and analyses possible solutions, while appreciative inquiry discusses what the future should be.
- Appreciative inquiry adopts innovative actions.

(Adapted from Cooperrider and Whitney 2005)

Asset mapping is a way of promoting effective equity-focused policies, by identifying and measuring community capacity, in order to promote health development activities (Morgan and Ziglio 2007). It is a process of assessing and recording the contributions people make to their communities, including their personal strengths and other resources that are available. This focuses on the assets of people as well as the physical and environmental aspects of place. It enables people to feel positive about where they live and the opportunities there can be for change. It is often considered the starting point for communities recognizing what is available to them, and how those assets can be utilized to enhance the environment and the services and contribute to improved health and well-being (Sigerson and Gruer 2011).

Essentially, a community asset is anything that improves the quality of community life. Assets include the knowledge and abilities of individuals, the physical buildings and places, the agencies that provide employment, including businesses, the public sector, the third sector, local groups, and public, private and community organizations (UCLA Center for Health Policy Research n.d.).

Social capital

Social capital can be defined as:

> the personal contacts and social networks that generate shared understandings, trust and reciprocity within and between social groups, and which underpin co-operation and collective action, the basis of economic prosperity and economic inclusion. Social capital can be accumulated when people interact in a purposeful manner with each other in families, workplaces, neighbourhoods, local associations and a range of informal and formal meeting places. (Miles *et al.* 2005, p.ii)

Benefits of social capital include improved confidence and self-esteem, a feeling of connectedness and belonging and a sense of self-efficacy and control (Edinburgh Health Inequalities Standing Group n.d.), all of which are proven protective factors in relation to health (Campbell, Wood and Kelly 1999).

Putnam (1993), working in the US and Italy, found some societies characterized by authoritarian, hierarchical, political and social relations. Other areas had more egalitarian social and political relations and were associated with more voluntary civic participation based on personal freedom. Research has consistently found that the latter kind of society is linked with good health outcomes, including reduced morbidity and mortality (Berkman and Kawachi 2000; Wilkinson 2005).

Putnam (1993) identified five key elements of social capital:

- community networks
- civic engagement
- local civic identity
- reciprocity between community members
- trust in the community.

Social capital has become a key concept in community development work. Both are built on mutual respect, trust and reciprocity and are concerned with developing relationships between people. However, it must be recognized that there can be a downside to social capital in that communities can be linked in an unbalanced way. It can divide communities, wherein some elements have strong connections to the detriment of those on the periphery of society. It can maintain barriers, through promoting exclusive networks or by creating and promoting strong bonds between antisocial groups, such as criminal or drug gangs (Portes 1998).

Social networks

The phrase 'social network' is a much used and often undefined phrase. One suggested definition is that it is 'the relationships that exist between groups of individuals or agencies, and the resources to which membership of such groups facilitates access' (Hawes, Webster and Sheill 2004, p.971).

Social networks have been found to be positively and consistently associated with morbidity and mortality (Berkman and Kawachi 2000). As well as improving physical health, social support can also improve mental health by offering opportunities for social interaction and help with practical problems, thereby reducing loneliness and improving levels of perceived support; by helping individuals cope with:

> the 'hassles' of everyday life by giving reassurance that the individual is loved and valued, which enhances self-esteem and feelings of self-worth; by giving reassurance and feedback about the individual's competence, thus helping to restore a sense of mastery and control. (Cooper *et al.* 1999, p.15)

A recent phenomenon is the development of social networking services. These services provide a platform, usually web based, to build social networks among people who share interests, activities, backgrounds or real-life connections. A social network service consists of a representation of each user (often a profile), his/her social links and a variety of additional services. Most social network services facilitate users to interact over the Internet, for example using email and instant messaging, and allow users to share ideas, pictures, posts, activities, events and interests with people in their network (Wikipedia contributors 2012).

The potential for social networking services to be pro-actively used to improve health and well-being has yet to be understood, although some examples are developing. For example, Netmums is a UK-based family of local websites set up and run by mothers. It includes a discussion forum and provides support and advice for parents on a national level, using advertising to generate revenue. Netmums has more than 1,500,000 members, approximately 4 million unique users a month and more than 27 million page views a month, making it the UK's most popular social networking, advice and support website (Wikipedia contributors 2013).

On the other hand there have been some high-profile examples of stress and even suicide caused by online bullying (see also Chapter 3). Websites such as that of ChildLine give advice to young people who are particularly likely to be victims of online bullying.

Co-production

Co-production is increasingly being seen as a central element to successful change in delivering services. There are many definitions of co-production, but it is generally acknowledged that engagement, choice and control, participation and involvement are all key aspects (DH 2010a). One definition agreed by service users and carers is that 'co-production is when you as an individual influence the support and services you receive, or when groups of people get together to influence the way that services are designed, commissioned and delivered' (Putting People First n.d., p.17). That definition focuses on services. Hanley (2013) suggests a more inclusive definition, emphasizing the importance of working with and from people's perspective, rather than that of the service providers:

> Co-production is an assets approach that builds on the skills, knowledge, experience, networks and resources that individuals and

communities bring. Built on equal relationships where individuals, families, communities and service providers have a reciprocal and equal relationship, an approach where services 'do with not to' the people who use them and who act as their own catalysts for change. (*ibid.*, p.14)

There are several reasons for the increased interest in co-production. It is being more widely recognized that markets or centralized bureaucracies are not the most effective or efficient ways of delivering public services based on relationships, such as those in health and social care. Personal services that are sensitive to individual need and are not concerned with profit need a different approach if they are to be useful. Empowering people and building on their social networks are of critical importance in delivering services from the users' perspective (Stephens, Ryan-Collins and Boyle 2008).

Capacity building

Capacity building has been defined as 'activities, resources and support that strengthen the skills, abilities and confidence of people and community groups to take effective action and leading roles in the development of communities' (Skinner 2006, cited in Scottish Community Development Centre for Learning Connections 2007, p.3).

Capacity building is important for community development, in that it is associated with adult and informal education, supporting collective action and developing specific outcomes. Evaluation of the New Deal for Communities programme in England has shown that, without empowerment of local residents, participation in decision making at both a practice and a policy level is unlikely to have a long-term impact. For this process to occur, capacity building, involving skill enhancement and personal development programmes, is essential (Batty *et al.* 2010).

To be effective, capacity building needs to 'focus on the community perspective, its needs and issues' (Scottish Community Development Centre for Learning Connections (SCDCLC) 2007, p.4). The SCDCLC stresses the need to make use of action-based research and to encourage, support or increase participation by and representation from the community (both individuals and groups). It recognizes also that different types of support are needed, for example training or planning advice.

Capacity building involves promoting participation in the local community and neighbourliness. It includes developing social networks, as well as work connections, and requires all the conditions relevant for community development, such as trust, reciprocity and cooperation. Action taken as a result of capacity building can lead to relatively straightforward achievements, such as parents working together with their local school to develop their skills as co-educators, through to complex interventions including lobbying ministers (Ferguson *et al.* 2008).

The principles of capacity building can be applied in organizations as well as communities, and ideally both aspects would be occurring at the same time, so that professionals are expecting and supporting a pro-active role from community members and vice versa. The approach has been well developed in New South Wales, Australia (NSW Health 2001): 'The rationale for capacity-building is simple. By building sustainable skills, resources and commitments to health promotion in health care settings, community settings and in other sectors, health promotion workers prolong and multiply health gains many times over' (Hawe *et al.* 2000, p.2).

This process of working at all levels of the organization to identify tackling inequalities and promoting mental health and well-being as part of its purpose, and therefore the role of staff, is sometimes referred to as 'making every contact count'.

The New South Wales Framework for Building Capacity to Improve Health identified five key areas for organizations to pay attention to in order to expand the number of people actively addressing inequalities in health, including mental health: organizational change, workforce development, resource allocation, partnerships and leadership (NSW Health 2001). Capacity building can include skills as diverse as canvassing, developing skills in negotiation, supporting policy, developing partnerships, understanding intelligence and using evidence. Change often progresses in stages: awareness, adoption, implementation and institutionalization of change.

The need to undertake capacity building across sectors has been recognized in the UK by the recent Healthy Lives, Healthy People Public Health Workforce Strategy (Public Health Policy and Strategy Unit 2013), in which the wider workforce involved in public health is described as follows:

It consists of a diverse range of professional groups currently working in the NHS, national and local government, academic departments and elsewhere who are performing a wide range of health and care functions. What unifies them in the first instance is a shared commitment to using their skills and experience to deliver public health outcomes across the three domains of public health: health improvement, health protection and healthcare public health. This strategy is also, in one way or another, for all of them. (*ibid.*, p.4)

One example of capacity building developed within the health service in England but reaching out to engage with the community is the Community Health Champions approach, developed by Altogether Better (NHS Confederation 2012). The aim is to develop a network of local people who work in partnership to promote health. They are individuals who are trained and supported to volunteer, to inspire and support their friends, neighbours, communities and work colleagues to live healthier lives, by making positive lifestyle changes. Evidence shows increased self-esteem and confidence, improvements in both physical and mental health, as well as increased awareness and knowledge of health issues (South, White and Woodall 2010). The return on investment for each £1 spent was up to £112.42 (Hex and Tatlock 2011).

DEVELOP PERSONAL SKILLS

In this section we address specific areas of personal skills development (including modifying harmful behaviours) that are relevant to mental health and well-being.

As covered in Chapters 2 and 4, some key aspects of emotional, cognitive and behavioural skill development occur during the first two years of a child's life, and some of the most effective interventions to address this issue rely on tackling the wider determinants of health, such as income. This material on interventions in early childhood is therefore not repeated here and this section focuses on adults. It is worth pointing out that much work with adults will also benefit children, for example working with parents of very young children may involve health literacy. Topics covered here flow from more generally applicable training and education through to more personal lifestyle choices.

Training to enhance self-esteem and self-confidence

There is a wide range of courses aimed at improving self-esteem and self-confidence, through the NHS, the local authority, the third sector and private business. Some examples are listed below:

- Stress management: this is a recognized approach to addressing stress in the workplace (NICE 2009d).

- Enhancing self-esteem and self-confidence: many courses are available, often based on the principles of cognitive behavioural therapy, whereby people are helped to understand their thoughts and feelings and how they influence their behaviour (IAPT n.d.).

- Mindfulness: there is a growing interest in the benefits of mindfulness, an approach that encourages the individual to be aware, observe without criticism and accept themselves for who they are. It is based on Buddhist teachings, and is practised through meditation, although it is not religious in content (Williams and Penman 2011). It is being applied to many aspects of chronic conditions management (Kabat-Zinn 2012).

- Assertiveness training: assertiveness training aims to give participants more confidence and directness in claiming their rights or putting forward their views, without falling back on unhelpful behaviour, which may be passive, aggressive or manipulative (Townend 2007). NICE recommends assertiveness training for looked-after children and young people experiencing bullying and violence. Such training is considered appropriate for promoting self-esteem and confidence, as well as enhancing well-being (NICE and SCIE 2010, modified April 2013). NICE further recognizes the importance for people with mental health problems of dealing assertively with staff. It is seen as a key element in the person-centred approach advocated in shared decision making around an individual's care (NICE 2011b).

Positive mental health and happiness networks

The New Economics Foundation (Aked et al. 2009) has suggested an approach to addressing positive mental health that involves focusing on promoting five areas of an individual's life that may enhance well-being.

These are:

- connecting: having strong social relationships
- being active: being physically active
- taking notice: being aware of what is around
- learning: being involved in learning
- giving: giving, sharing with others.

These activities have been shown to have a sound evidence base to promoting health and well-being, as well as having the potential to reduce the number of people developing mental health problems.

An example of a similar approach being used at a local level is Tameside and Glossop's high-profile campaign encouraging people to incorporate the 'five ways to well-being' into their lives (Tameside and Glossop Clinical Commissioning Group 2012).

Action for Happiness is a movement for positive social change, identifying ten keys to happiness, along the same lines to the five quoted above.

> For fifty years we've aimed relentlessly at higher incomes. But despite being much wealthier, we're no happier than we were five decades ago. At the same time we've seen an increase in wider social issues, including a worrying rise in anxiety and depression in young people. It's time for a positive change in what we mean by progress. (Action for Happiness 2013)

A possible criticism of the movement is that it does not adequately acknowledge the social and economic determinants of health, which cannot be side-stepped by aspiring to a less materialistic culture (although this in itself may be a worthwhile goal). However, it aims to publicize the known differences in resilience among both individuals and populations, and seeks to use these differences for social benefit.

Health literacy

Health promotion, and in particular mental health promotion, supports:

> personal and social development through providing information, education for health, and enhancing life skills. By so doing, it increases the options available to people to exercise more control

over their own health and over their environments, and to make choices conducive to health. (WHO 2009a, p.3)

A key element of the role of education in health promotion is health literacy. This includes supporting people to develop a whole range of skills related to health information – reading, obtaining and interpreting it, be it on paper or electronic and in words or in the form of graphs. Examples include information about prescriptions, medical test results or local health services (Glassman 2013).

There are many approaches to improving health literacy, many using a community development approach, supporting individuals and communities to understand health information in the broadest sense (Nutbeam 2000). Schools have been identified as a key setting to promote health literacy (St Leger 2001). Hospital settings have also been used, for example, with Skilled for Health courses (developed jointly by the Department of Health and the Department for Education and Skills), aimed at improving knowledge of nutrition among hospital staff. In a pilot project in an acute hospital, course participants felt healthier and sometimes happier with themselves (often because of associated weight loss) (Brown 2009).

Continuing education

Not only health literacy but lifelong education can benefit mental well-being. Beyond the school years, continued formal and informal learning, as well as higher levels of qualifications, are associated with greater subjective well-being for individuals (APHO 2007; Hammond and Feinstein 2006; ONS 2012b).

Healthy lifestyle choices

As discussed in Chapter 4, many behaviours can adversely affect mental as well as physical health. Interventions that help people to moderate these behaviours therefore potentially enhance mental well-being, as described in the following subsections. Many interventions involve the behaviour change model discussed in Chapter 5.

Healthy eating

The relationship between physical health and mental health was discussed in Chapter 4. Eating sensibly can improve physical health and reduce obesity (a factor contributing to depression). However, there are also direct effects on mental health. For example, it has been shown that children who regularly eat breakfast have better concentration, are more alert and miss fewer days of school (e.g. Mayo Clinic 2014).

Physical activity

Group physical activity programmes are recommended for people with mild to moderate depression (NCCMH 2009). Evidence shows that all intensity levels of exercise can contribute to psychological well-being, and longer-term programmes can be more effective. All types of activity have been found helpful, with choice being a key element. Whitelaw *et al.* (2008) did find some evidence around the type of exercise: for example, activities such as weight resistance training improved body image and self-esteem; group recreational sports improved mood; and cooperative exercise settings produced stronger effects.

Alcohol, smoking and substance misuse

NICE Guidelines (NICE 2010) and the government's Alcohol Strategy (HM Government 2012c) recognize a range of approaches to reducing alcohol-related harm, including pricing, reducing access by children and young people, restricting advertising, educating people about it and providing brief interventions for people at risk of becoming dependent.

Evidence suggests that about half of smokers with a mental health problem wish to quit smoking but 'stop smoking' services are not routinely offered to this group. A range of services has been shown to be effective, including psychological and lifestyle approaches, cognitive behavioural therapy and nicotine replacement therapy, although some medications can affect and be affected by smoking (Campion, Checinski and Nurse 2008).

The government's drug strategy (HM Government 2010a) emphasizes the importance of breaking intergenerational paths of drug dependency by providing support to vulnerable families, for example through the Family Nurse Partnership programme, to provide good-quality advice and credible information to actively resist misusing drugs. Encouraging people to take responsibility for their own health and providing early intervention is seen as important. The recent All Party Parliamentary Group for Drug Policy Reform (2013) report provides evidence to suggest that decriminalization of drugs (rather than banning drugs) may reduce crime, homelessness, unemployment and relationship problems.

Sexual health

In many ways, promoting good sexual health in young people requires the same approaches as promoting good general mental health to this group, such as providing positive parental involvement, promoting self-esteem and self-confidence in young people (Trivedi *et al.* 2007). A related intervention is around conduct disorder and violent behaviour (Barlow *et al.* 2007).

CREATE SUPPORTIVE ENVIRONMENTS

This is the fourth of the Ottawa Charter areas for action. In Chapter 5 we looked at the strategic need to understand decisions about the use of resources of all kinds, including the workforce. Practical examples are provided in this section.

The links between mental health and inequalities in health measured by life expectancy and chronic illness are very strong. There is a wide range of evidence showing that mental well-being has an impact on the inequalities that affect health (Friedli 2009). Tackling inequalities means doing more to create socially just environments. Examples of the way this can happen are included below, where we consider particular at-risk groups before moving on to a discussion of the way a settings approach can be used to enhance mental well-being.

In Chapters 2, 3 and 4 the main factors affecting people's mental health were outlined. In this section we present some of the interventions that have been shown to be effective in addressing those factors. This list matches that in Chapter 3 as well as the evidence permits, although interventions relating to BME groups and those with long-term conditions are covered instead in the relevant case studies. Where evidence is available, headings from Chapters 2 and 4 are also included.

Bereavement

NICE (2004a) suggests that although most people have sufficient personal resources to deal with bereavement, offering additional support to some people may be important. This may be around practical, financial, social, spiritual and emotional needs, and could include providing information or more focused support around the emotional and psychological impact of bereavement. A range of self-help groups, counselling services and other forms of Third Sector provision can provide the help that may be needed. For young people, there is a website set up by Cruse where people can share experiences and feelings.

Bullying

We outline measures around bullying in later 'settings' subsections, considering schools and workplaces. The issue is also discussed in the case study chapters.

Carers

Several areas need to be addressed to improve the experiences of carers (DH 2010b). First is the need to support carers in identifying themselves as such early on, in order to involve them in developing local provision and planning care packages. Also emphasized is the importance of enabling carers to fulfil their potential in terms of education and employment.

Deprivation and poverty

The strain imposed by financial difficulties was highlighted in Chapter 2. It has been found that specialist welfare advice can cut the cost of mental health care in three main ways: reductions in inpatient lengths of stay, prevention of homelessness, and prevention of relapse (Lewis 2013). It is recognized that those in financial difficulty may feel too ashamed or scared to ask for help, so usually the services recommended by organizations are those that are not judgemental (Mind n.d. a).

Homelessness

The Mental Health Foundation (2002) suggested several ways to improve mental health in homeless young people, including:

- better provision of supported accommodation and half-way houses
- more education and active health promotion for young people around mental health issues
- improved accessibility to preventive and primary care services
- improved family mediation and respite services, including befriending, mentoring and peer support
- better education and training for key professional groups (health and social care, crime and housing) on mental health issues.

The government has expressed a commitment (e.g. DCLG 2012a) to improve outcomes for homeless people with dual drugs/alcohol and mental health needs, and to ensure medical professionals discharging patients know where to go for help in meeting housing needs.

Looked-after children

NICE guidance on looked-after children (NICE and SCIE 2010, modified April 2013) stresses the need for good record-keeping, for improved education and for dedicated services to promote mental health and well-being, particularly where the children are being placed out of a local authority area and risk not receiving CAMH (Child and Adolescent Mental Health) services in the new location.

The NSPCC (2011, section 6) stresses the need for ensuring the safety of looked-after children and stresses that 'the experience of all children and young people placed in the care system in the UK should be positive and of good quality'.

Offenders

Measures to be taken include having effective strategies to reduce bullying and violence, identification and protection of particularly vulnerable prisoners (vulnerable either because of their offence or because of personal circumstances), risk assessments around cell-sharing and monitoring of incidents. Ensuring adequate assessment in prison and appropriate continuity of care on release is essential in making sure this group's health issues are addressed (NEPHO 2005).

People with learning disabilities

There should be regular health checks and good liaison across services. Family carers and people with learning disabilities themselves should be involved in all decisions about their care at all stages (Michael 2008).

Refugees and asylum-seekers

Improving the processes for refugees and asylum-seekers, and particularly reducing the length of time they spend in detention, can help to ensure that the system does not add to the stress already caused by the circumstances of their becoming refugees or asylum-seekers.

Counselling services are needed, as for any group, but, because there can be difficulties maintaining contact, a multi-agency coordinated approach is important. There may also be difficulties in persuading refugees to accept counselling if it is not a familiar concept in their own culture and, if it is accepted, refugees may be anxious about revealing any personal information (Tribe 2002). Among other helpful approaches is ensuring that front-line staff are familiar with the issues surrounding refugees and other migrants (Rodger and Chappel 2008).

Sexual abuse and sexual exploitation

Women who are experiencing domestic violence approach health services more frequently than women who are not (Ratner 1993). SSIA (2011) stressed that all staff who come into contact with women should be appropriately trained to identify signs of domestic violence and be aware of what action should be taken.

Counselling can be helpful to victims of sexual abuse. Children and young people with post-traumatic stress disorder, including those who have been sexually abused, should be offered trauma-focused cognitive behavioural therapy, adapted appropriately to suit their age, circumstances and levels of development. Adults may also need drug treatment alongside cognitive behavioural therapy (NICE 2005). Female genital mutilation is discussed in Chapter 8.

There are mixed outcomes from approaches to treating perpetrators to reduce domestic abuse. Completing a course for perpetrators may stop violence for a period, but it may be replaced by verbal or psychological abuse (Romans, Poore and Martin 2000). Schemes to address co-occurring alcohol dependence and perpetration of intimate partner violence work for some participants, but others may need longer-term or more intensive treatment (Oberleitner, Mandel and Easton 2013). Programmes to reduce intimate partner violence have been found to be successful for adolescents, but these may not be equally effective in other groups or contexts (De Grace and Clarke 2012).

Sexuality

Mainstream services need to be aware of the lesbian, gay, bisexual and transgender (LGBT) population and be sensitive to their needs. This will require: training in LGBT issues for all mainstream services; ensuring the LGBT population have equal access to services; appropriate sign-posting; inclusion of appropriate images of LGBT people in all literature; and the promotion of hate crime reporting systems, with responses reviewed on a regular basis to inform action (Ash and Mackereth 2013).

Social isolation and inclusion

Older people are at risk of social isolation, and evidence suggests that addressing social isolation can be an effective way to improve mental well-being (Mackereth and Appleton 2008). Critical to this is the provision of services that engage people in activities with other people. Effective interventions include mentoring and involvement with social group schemes and self-help (SCIE 2011). Other interventions that have proved positive in addressing loneliness include group activities with an education or support element, particularly when targeted at specific groups, and physical activity interventions (Cattan et al. 2005). The Mental Health Foundation (2010b) emphasizes the need for organizations providing services to ensure that the physical environment is not off-putting to older men (for example, organizations should consider the décor, the music and facilities such as a clearly marked male toilet).

Being able to continue living independently is also important for the emotional well-being of older people, and this can be helped by some of the activities that address social isolation, such as the provision of good public transport (and free bus passes and discounted rail travel).

Veterans of the armed services

Veteran support organizations in the third sector, along with the Ministry of Defence, can address the emotional and practical support needs of those returning to civilian life. In recent years there has been a wider range of cross-government support (HM Government, 2008).

Victims and survivors of domestic violence

A range of interventions is needed to address the issues. Apart from the treatment of victims, which may involve counselling, a key element is getting front-line services to recognize the problems. There is also a need not only to punish offenders but to take preventive measures to reduce the risk of re-offending. The government is now adopting a zero tolerance approach to violence or abuse in the family (Home Office 2013b) and has created professional guidance for health visitors and school nursing programmes (DH 2013b). There are also 'sanctuary schemes' that are aimed at helping people in households at risk of domestic violence to stay in their homes (DCLG 2010).

Settings work

In Chapter 5 we discussed the high-level impact of decisions on the physical environment where people live, work and play. For organizations or practitioners these may seem far removed from day-to-day life. However, service planners may make use of a 'settings' approach to help them to think about creating change through targeting the organizations and their social systems that shape individual behaviour. Settings work is based on thinking about the whole system (Grossman and Scala 1993).

While the previous subsections considered ways of reaching particular at-risk groups of individuals, an advantage of settings work is that it potentially reaches everyone in the setting, giving access to different at-risk groups. The sequence is to work from the widest settings – the natural and local environment, via the built environment (cities and housing), through to more specific settings where adults work or young people attend pre-school or education.

Healthy and safe environment

National and local government can promote more sustainable lifestyles, some of which affect health very directly, such as providing good pedestrian and cycle access to services and encouraging the use of public transport (and supporting its development). Modelling studies suggest that active travel strategies can reduce rates of depression (FPH 2013). Planners can also plan the spatial environment so that it is conducive to health, for example encouraging physical activity, maintaining a sense of safety and using water and vegetation to create a natural 'feel'.

The range of beneficial activities associated with outdoor exercise is very wide, including such things as mentioned by Mind (2013) in its discussion of ecotherapy: conservation or farm activities, art-based activities using natural materials and contact with animals. Ecotherapy (in its strict sense) is about building a relationship with nature, so that personal well-being is considered equally alongside the health of the environment. Ecotherapy sessions usually include some type of formal therapy, such as cognitive behavioural therapy or counselling, and reportedly reduce depression and improve mental well-being (*ibid.*).

There are roles for many other local authority departments. Environmental health departments can act to reduce noise nuisance or other environmental factors contributing to stress. Trading standards departments can strengthen action to prevent young people accessing tobacco or alcohol.

Another aspect of a healthy environment is crime levels, with the potential adverse effects of crime on mental health as mentioned in Chapter 2. The Home Office (2013a) has identified a number of areas to focus on to prevent crime. A key element is responding to antisocial behaviour, which includes helping agencies to identify and support high-risk victims, giving professionals on the front line more autonomy and improving understanding of the experiences of victims (Home Office 2012). Community safety partnerships, which are multi-agency, are expected to be used more to work out local approaches to problems.

Healthy cities

The WHO Healthy Cities global movement engages local governments in health development through a process of political commitment, institutional change, capacity building, partnership-based planning and innovative projects.

The primary goal of the WHO European Healthy Cities Network (WHO Regional Office for Europe n.d.) is to put health high on the social, economic and political agendas of city governments. Health is the business of all sectors, and local governments are in a unique leadership position, with power to protect and promote their citizens' health and well-being. The Healthy Cities movement promotes comprehensive and systematic policy and planning for health and emphasizes:

- the need to address inequality in health and urban poverty
- the needs of vulnerable groups
- participatory governance
- the social, economic and environmental determinants of health.

Many practical steps can be taken. For example, town planners should ensure that new traffic systems do not split communities or lead to isolation. Accessible green space should also be provided. Councils can provide cultural and leisure services, including libraries, galleries and museums, which support meaningful physical and social activities.

Healthy housing

With housing also, relatively straightforward interventions can significantly improve mental well-being. For example, maintaining investment in affordable public housing, to protect those who cannot maintain mortgages (and their dependants) from becoming homeless, impacts on mental health by reducing anxiety and poor health-related behaviour among those who fear they may be about to lose their job (Stuckler and Basu 2013). Support with housing can improve people's mental health and can help reduce the demand overall for health and social care services (Bolton 2009).

Help available around housing to those with mental health problems includes:

- outreach support to help people stay in their own homes
- short-stay hostels, supported flats and group homes, respite care and residential care homes
- crisis houses (with short-term support to help resolve crises without hospital admission)
- therapeutic communities – similar to supported flats, but normally they put a greater emphasis on rehabilitation. They are

places where social relationships, the structure of the day and different group activities are all deliberately designed to help health and well-being.

(Mind n.d. b)

Practical help with housing can also enable older people to continue living independently, helping their emotional well-being. Simply installing handrails to allow an older infirm person to feel safe about going outside the home can reduce the chance of them becoming socially isolated (Brown 2012).

Healthy workplaces

Workplace health has received increasing government attention in recent years. In England, Dame Carol Black emphasized the need to help people to find and stay in work, noting that the stigma around ill health needed to be tackled. This was particularly true for those with mental health problems, where employers do not always realize how much they can help.

The workplace can be a good way of reaching those who are in paid employment, and may be helpful in targeting the very low paid or those with low self-esteem. Black's review stressed the need for employers to take action to improve health and well-being, in particular mentioning the positive effects of psychosocial therapies on people's ability to work. It also stressed the need for preventive action and promotion of well-being in the workplace. This was then reflected in NICE guidance on promoting mental health at work: recommendations include a strategic and coordinated approach to promoting employees' mental well-being and, where feasible, flexible working, which 'can enhance employees' sense of control and promote engagement and job satisfaction' (NICE 2009d, p.10).

A whole variety of issues affect health in the workplace environment, many with a direct or indirect link with mental health:

- food in the canteen or dining room, policy on snacks available, eating/kitchen areas for packed lunches
- corporate approach to stress
- employee welfare programmes that address alcohol and drug use
- proactive employment of people who have or have had mental health problems

- access to occupational health.

(NICE 2009c)

Healthy workplaces have been endorsed by the UK Responsibility Deal. The core commitment, 'We will actively support our workforce to lead healthier lives', provides a framework for the work of the network, which has developed a number of pledges that organizations can sign up to. For example, the pledge related to mental health includes:

> We will create an environment where anyone with past or present experience of mental health issues is valued, respected and able to flourish. This will involve providing all staff with the environment, knowledge and tools to develop and maintain emotional resilience and mental wellbeing, while raising awareness of, and providing support for, mental health in the workplace. (DH n.d. b)

Healthy pre-school settings and parenting

Barlow *et al.* (2007) identified a variety of programmes that were effective in promoting mental health and preventing mental health problems in children and young people. Parenting programmes were found to be the most effective, followed by interventions for conduct disorder and violence prevention, and self-esteem programmes.

The Healthy Child Programme (Shribman and Billingham 2009) provides a comprehensive programme of developmental reviews and health promotion programmes, including information and guidance to support parenting. This is an evidence-based programme offered to all families with pre-school children. In many areas, it is supplemented by the Family Nurse Partnership, a programme offering intensive, structured home visiting to young families (Family Nurse Partnership National Unit 2012).

Healthy schools

The PSHE (personal, social and health education) curriculum is important in promoting health and well-being to children, which can affect their well-being throughout life. School can also be an accessible setting for much work around mental well-being. Some benefits will accrue from initiatives designed primarily for physical health, such as breakfast clubs or football clubs (the benefits to mental health of physical exercise and food were mentioned earlier).

As England's Healthy Schools Programme developed, following its launch in 1999, it laid greater stress on emotional health and well-being. More than half of the coordinators in both primary and secondary schools felt the programme had helped this (NatCen 2011). One element of success appears to have been the way the programme raised awareness of the issues.

The Department for Education website includes a healthy schools toolkit (DfE n.d.). One example it presents is of a successful whole-school programme in Barnsley to reduce alcohol consumption, among families at risk, working with the local child and adolescent mental health service. Evaluation suggests that this intervention may have worked well because it:

- adopts a whole-school approach
- develops behavioural approaches with life skills
- adopts an interactive approach
- delivers over time, not a one off
- starts at a young age
- is led by trained individuals.

Supportive school environments, including access to health care professionals at school, are important protective factors among adolescents, including those who have experienced bullying, those with learning disabilities and those with ADHD (The Scottish Government 2004).

The reduction of bullying in schools is helped by the implementation of bullying policies in schools. As part of the Healthy Schools programme in England, some schools began to log and report occurrences of bullying and discrimination (NatCen 2011). Teachers can receive awareness-raising training.

Tackling truancy is also essential, and the government-commissioned report on school attendance (C. Taylor 2012) presents recommendations that include primary schools making better use of data on absence and focusing on vulnerable pupils, and the use of parental sanctions. The government's Troubled Families Programme, although targeting only a very small number of families with multiple problems, has also reported some success in reducing truancy (DCLG 2012b).

REORIENTATE SERVICES

This is the fifth action area of the Ottawa Charter strategic plan to create health and well-being. A key part of it suggested that the health sector must move beyond curative services. Programmes have been found to use a mixture of activities, including: exercise on referral; arts on prescription; community education groups; self-help groups or resources; computerized cognitive behavioural therapy; bibliotherapy; group activities on referral; time banks (schemes that enable people to exchange skills with one another, with a log of time spent); and volunteering (Johnson and Ross 2011).

Most of the NICE recommendations relating to acute secondary care services apply equally to mental health services and are stressed in all mental health-related NICE guidance (e.g. NCCMH 2011c). These include: ensuring equal access for those with learning disability; ensuring equal access for BME groups and providing culturally appropriate services, with translation if needed; treating with respect all patients, including those who self-harm; ensuring that users and carers are involved in service development; and age-appropriate admissions for children and adolescents.

This section considers several practical ways that mental health services can be improved: social prescribing; health improvement and wellness services; and dealing with depression. It then focuses on the practical implications of involving users and carers, which, as indicated in Chapter 5, is a key lever in work to reorientate services. Then it considers the issues around integration of services. It concludes with a discussion of two review tools – Health Equity Audit and evaluation.

Social prescribing

Social prescribing is a mechanism for linking people with non-medical activities or sources of support within the community (Friedli *et al.* 2009). It offers alternatives to clinical provision or medication, such as information, support and activities (such as volunteering or physical activity). It is sometimes called community referral and was developed initially for people with mild to moderate mental health problems.

Social prescribing has been shown to provide a range of positive outcomes, including cognitive, emotional and social benefits, and is part of a wider recognition of the influence of social and cultural factors on mental health outcomes (Brown, Friedli and Watson 2004). Both short-term and long-term benefits have been identified (Friedli *et al.* 2009), affecting health services provision, social inclusion and awareness of mental health improvement measures. Benefits to health service provision include reductions in the length of waiting lists for psychological services, reductions in antidepressant prescribing levels and reductions in the numbers of people attending services frequently (*ibid.*). Increasing numbers of people (including socially isolated people and clients of mental health services) take advantage of activities such as arts or leisure, so that social isolation is reduced (*ibid.*). There is also an 'increased awareness of skills, activities and behaviours that improve and protect mental well-being – e.g. the adoption of positive steps for mental health' (*ibid.*, p.7).

Health improvement and wellness services

Health improvement services have historically been commissioned to address behaviour change using the behaviour change model, addressing one aspect of lifestyle at a time, such as smoking, weight or use of alcohol. However, a report by the King's Fund (Buck and Frosini 2012) looked at how these behaviours clustered together in the population and how multiple lifestyle risk patterns had changed between different population groups in the period 2003–2008. They found that the overall proportion of the population engaging in three or four of four unhealthy behaviours – smoking, excessive alcohol use, poor diet, and low levels of physical activity – had declined significantly. However, the reductions had been seen mainly among those in higher socio-economic and educational groups: people with no qualifications were more than five times as likely as those with higher education to engage in all four poor behaviours in 2008, compared with being only three times as likely in 2003. The report recommended a holistic approach to policy and practice that addresses lifestyles encompassing multiple unhealthy behaviours.

One developing approach is to create a wellness service that includes mental well-being. A wellness service 'provides support to people in order to improve their health and well-being. The service aims to build people's capacity to live healthy lives by addressing the factors that influence health and wellbeing' (NHS Confederation 2011, p.1). In this way, one integrated service has the potential to address the interaction of lifestyle issues that particularly affect the most disadvantaged. Services specifically addressing health-related issues such as smoking, weight management and drinking are offered in a broader context.

A review of the evidence related to the impact of wellness services found many benefits to users, including:

- promotion of positive health that can empower individuals, enabling them to maintain and improve their own health
- provision of safe, natural means to boost physical and mental health without unpleasant side effects
- facilitation of lifestyle adjustments to enable individuals to gain wellness
- a focus on promoting quality of life, not just length of life
- enhanced self-esteem, improved mood and greater confidence
- improved self-management of a long-term health condition and helping people to return to work.

(Adapted from Winters *et al.* 2010, p.62)

As an example of an integrated approach to health and well-being reaching out to the community, the Southern Health and Social Care Trust created a promoting well-being team, an 'integrated team leading on the planning and delivery of approaches to improve health and well-being and reduce health inequality across the area' (Public Health Agency 2010, p.16). Community development was recognized as central to this approach, which helped to dovetail plans with the health and well-being work of other organizations in the area.

Diagnosing and dealing with depression

A formal diagnosis of depression requires a person to report low mood, loss of interest and pleasure or loss of energy on most days over the previous two weeks (NICE 2009a). If a practitioner suspects depression it is appropriate to ask two questions. The first is a direct question about feelings of depression: 'During the last month, have you often been bothered by feeling down, depressed or hopeless?' (*ibid.*, 1.3.1.1). The second is concerned with any lack of interest or pleasure that the patient might be experiencing (another key indicator of depression): 'During the last month, have you often been bothered by having little interest or pleasure in doing things?' (*ibid.*) If the answer to either of these questions is 'yes', the patient should be given or referred for a mental health assessment.

At the mild end of the depression spectrum, there are clear links with the promotion of good mental health. Many health improvement programmes focus at this level, and would include a wide range of self-help groups, including assertiveness training and courses to enhance self-esteem and self-confidence, social prescribing and volunteering.

Front-line health and social services staff may not always be aware of the increased risks to mental health found in particular groups of people, including socially isolated people or people in certain family structures (as mentioned in Chapter 3). Despite the prevalence of mental ill health in the older population attending the GP surgery, only 3 per cent of practice nurses have received any mental health training (Age Concern 2007). Other groups for which opportunities to diagnose depression present themselves include:

- antenatal and post-natal women – health professionals should use a woman's first contacts with pre-birth and post-birth services to recognize the predictors of depression (NICE 2007)
- people with dual diagnosis – a more holistic approach is needed (Hughes 2006), for example training alcohol service workers at least to recognize common mental health problems
- veterans of the armed services – the government-commissioned Murrison Report recommendations included mental health assessments (Murrison 2010).

In line with the stepped-care model mentioned in Chapter 5, NICE guidelines (NCCMH 2011c) advise that antidepressants should not be used as a first-line treatment for mild depression. However, there may seem to be few alternatives available. The Mental Health Foundation found that 78 per cent of GPs have prescribed an antidepressant despite their belief that an alternative approach may have been more appropriate, and, of these, 66 per cent have done so because a suitable alternative was not available (Halliwell 2005).

Service user and carer involvement

Particularly where mental health services are concerned, not only the service users but their families and carers also need to be considered. As Wales's mental health strategy (Welsh Government 2012) says, 'families and carers of all ages, especially young carers, have an important role in the care and treatment of people with mental health problems' (p.32).

There are many advantages in involving service users and carers:

- They are experts in their experience and knowledge of services.
- They have their own perspectives that can challenge providers, and enable them to re-evaluate services.
- Decisions will be seen in a more positive light by other users and carers.
- There is improved design, and services are more effective and better value.
- Involvement can itself improve health and well-being.

(Husband, Carr and Jepson 2010)

Organizational change can be aided by various tools. The 'lean thinking' method has recently been applied to the public sector (Seddon 2012). It consists of clarifying the purpose of the service/system, and listening carefully to the nature of user demands. The change instigator then investigates the actual delivery, flow of work and underlying assumptions. Wasteful steps are removed or minimized, and the focus is on effective delivery, related to the users' experiences.

There are many techniques for involving service users and carers, often similar to those used to engage local people from a community development perspective. The choice of technique will depend on the purpose of the activity. Repper *et al.* (2011) identify some core principles for involving carers and users in research, which might be equally appropriate in other activities. These include respecting personal rights, being sensitive, making clear what is expected, being inclusive and providing resources.

Integrated care

Most sets of NICE recommendations emphasize the need for integrated care, for example in terms of clear pathways for patients and sharing of plans and information, particularly when a patient is transferring from one care setting to another. There are, however, problems associated with this: information sharing is governed by the need for confidentiality, so that it is not always possible to pass all relevant facts from one agency to another. Information-sharing protocols often have to be devised in order to cope with this.

The need for integrated care has been identified not just in general but for specific circumstances. A notable example is that of services for people with dual diagnosis, as mentioned in Chapter 4. The two services for people with alcohol or drug problems have not always been equipped to address mental health problems, while services for people with mental illness are not always prepared to address alcohol or drug issues. Services have different expertise and it has sometimes been difficult for them to work together to address these often strongly linked problems.

There are situations where specific integration of services is already happening. For instance, liaison psychiatry services provide a link between acute hospitals and psychiatric services, perhaps assessing risk in patients admitted to accident and emergency (A&E) departments and ensuring appropriate treatment or referral to further specialist treatment. Similarly, in some police stations, a mental health worker is available to assess those coming into custody. However, fully integrated services should be far wider than this, involving all agencies along the pathway that may be taken by a patient. This could mean health services (primary and secondary), social services, criminal justice services and third-sector organizations.

Easy access to services, with clear pathways, has been found to be important for many groups of people. For young people, access to mental health services should be via both health and education sectors (DH 2011b).

Good communication among relevant agencies (usually health care and social care) is also recommended, for example in keeping a service user's GP informed of plans (NCCMH 2004c) and recording and sharing plans for transition to another service (NCCMH 2012b).

Health Equity Audit

A measure that may be particularly useful to practitioners and organizations seeking to reorientate their service is a Health Equity Audit (HEA). This identifies how fairly services or other resources are distributed in relation to the health needs of different groups and areas, and prioritizes action required to provide services in relation to need. Actions required to create more equitable services (thereby reducing inequalities) are agreed and incorporated into local plans and practice. The overall aim is to distribute resources not equally, but in relation to health need (DH 2003).

One of the first activities with HEA is to produce an equity profile. This involves identifying the most common equity dimensions, including age, disability, gender reassignment, marriage and civil partnership, pregnancy and maternity, race, religion and belief, sex and sexual orientation. Service managers may be able to identify other dimensions of equity specifically relevant to their service. Then comes the collection of data to review the needs and the use of services by people in groups with those characteristics, with a view to comparing them with the wider population.

Hamer *et al.* (2006) describe the steps in the audit as a cycle. It starts with agreeing who is going to be involved inside and outside the organization, what the issue to be investigated in terms of equity is, and what the indicators may be. The next step is to compare service delivery across different groups in the population, compared with a profile of the population being served. The next two steps are identifying what local actions would make a difference, and then prioritizing them. Implementation usually involves some changes in resources and/or delivery. The final step in the cycle is reviewing service usage to see if there has been a changed pattern in favour of those with previously unmet needs.

Hamer *et al.* cite an example of a mental health services audit that identified the need for further investigation into the higher rates of hospital admissions in one deprived ward (particularly during holiday periods) and the disproportionate number of males and people from BME communities admitted under the Mental Health Act 1983.

Studies have considered inequity in access to services potentially caused by whether someone lives in an urban or a rural setting. Several factors have been found to affect service use or access in rural areas:

- If someone is prevented from driving because of a mental health problem, this might reduce the opportunities they have to access services (as well as increasing the likelihood of them becoming socially isolated).
- There might be a rural culture of stoicism, so that people are reluctant to seek help.
- People do not want to lose work time travelling to services.

- Anonymity and confidentiality are more difficult to guarantee in a small community.
- Stigma can be a real problem in a small community.

(Based on Nicholson 2008)

Evaluation

Another useful measure for service reorientation is evaluation, which should be applied to services that are genuinely innovative. The decision to evaluate should be made with the involvement of funders and other stakeholders at the start of the process. Evaluation requires the following steps:

1. Engage stakeholders (e.g. funders, collaborators, beneficiaries, elected members, primary users).

2. Describe the programme (What is its purpose? What changes may it realistically make to individual or organizational knowledge/attitudes/behaviour? What are ways the intervention is expected to make an impact?).

3. Focus the evaluation design in relation to its purpose (Is it to gain insight? to change practice? to assess effects? to affect participants?).

4. Gather evidence in relation to agreed indicators that reflect the purpose of the evaluation and the programme, using appropriate methods, for example surveys, documentation review, observation, focus groups and case studies.

5. Justify conclusions (interpret significance, make judgements according to clearly stated values, comparing results, consider alternative explanations, recommend decisions that are consistent with the conclusions).

6. Ensure use and share lessons learned (with planning, good communication and technical and emotional support, especially important in relation to negative findings).

(Adapted from Aceijas 2011, pp.114–124)

Evaluation of health gain, that is, the outcomes for the health of the population, is usually beyond the scope of an evaluation of a single service. Outcomes are a useful focus, but not a practical tool for service improvement (Seddon 2012).

The evaluation of the social, economic and environmental value of activities and interventions (social return on investment) was described in Chapter 1 and provides another approach to measuring success. 'Realistic evaluation' can add academic credibility to evaluation processes, using evaluators, planners and workers to establish:

- clarity in defining why the programme has the potential to cause change, and what the causal mechanisms for this may be
- understanding of the context and mechanisms underlying changed outcomes
- acknowledgement of the changing and permeable social world, where effectiveness can be enhanced or subverted through unanticipated intrusion of new contexts and causes.

(Adapted from Davies, Nutley and Smith 2000)

PRINCIPLES INTO PRACTICE

This chapter has again made use of the four principles for work related to mental health and well-being, with a focus on organizations and practitioners. In order to address the breadth of factors that enhance mental health and well-being (social, economic, cultural and environmental determinants), we need to involve capacity building across all settings. This is in line with our first and second principles that mental health and well-being is a holistic concept and that the 'determinants of health' must be addressed. Asset-based approaches are valuable to strengthen community action. Happiness networks focus on personal lifestyle and are a useful challenge to a commercially orientated society. However, neither approach will necessarily challenge structural inequalities. Reorientating health services involves central involvement of users and carers (part of our fourth principle), and may include integrated wellness services that are able to address 'clusters' of conditions. Health Equity Audit is a tool that providers can use to make sure their services are reaching those most in need. Evaluation of innovative services is important to build evidence from the front line, but in most cases using health care needs assessment and systematically assessed evidence about what works (our third principle) would, on its own, make a big difference to the effectiveness of delivery.

Chapter 7

EXTENDED CASE STUDY

PREVENTION OF SUICIDE AND SELF-HARM

KEY POINTS

- Suicide is committed by relatively small numbers of people, but with major impact on family, carers, friends and colleagues: it ranks in the top ten causes of death among young people.
- There are several issues about the measurement of suicide and self-harm, but there is an overall downward trend in the number of suicides.
- Those at higher risk of suicide include:
  - men
  - young people
  - people aged over 85.
- Life circumstances associated with depression are also likely to be linked to suicide.
- People already in contact with mental health services are a high-risk group, although numbers of suicides among them have been successfully reduced.
- Wider determinants that are particularly relevant include the economic situation, and education.
- The means of suicide is an important consideration in relation to prevention.
- Community-based interventions are relevant both for those at high risk, and more generically.

- A prevention strategy involves a very wide range of agencies, including the criminal justice system, planning authorities and schools, and these are identified as part of creating a supportive environment.
- Reorientating health services includes working across the health and social care system to reduce the risk of suicide.
- Suicide audit is a good example of a tool that can improve practice.

INTRODUCTION

We have chosen to carry out an extended case study on suicide because of its severity, and because the nature of the issue demands a whole-system approach. In this chapter, we consider the factors contributing to suicide and the various approaches that can be taken to understand the issues and help to prevent suicide. We outline interventions and activities that can help to prevent suicide, many of which also help to prevent self-harm, and we consider how to measure the quality of services and their impact on suicide prevention.

This is the first of three extended case studies. The sequence of headings from Chapter 2 (wider determinants), Chapter 4 (across the lifespan and personal behaviours) and Chapter 3 (life circumstances) is used wherever relevant. The final part of the case study uses the headings shared by Chapters 5 and 6 to discuss effective interventions.

THE IMPACT OF SUICIDE

As discussed in Chapter 1, the numbers of people who die by suicide are small in comparison with many other causes of death (some 6000 deaths per year in the UK). Nevertheless, suicide is a major public health issue, among the leading causes of death in certain age groups (see 'Across the lifespan' below). The effects of a suicide go far wider than the victim, as mentioned in Chapter 4.

Estimates have been made of the total cost of suicide per case (Johnson 2011), based on direct costs (services used before and following suicide), indirect costs (time lost from work and lost production) and human costs (years of disability-free life lost, pain and grief of families). The estimated average cost per case was £1.5 million in 2009 (*ibid.*).

DEFINITIONS

In discussing suicide, government statistics and policy-makers tend to include all deaths where the coroner's verdict was 'suicide' (where the victim intended death), 'injury undetermined' (where the victim's intentions were uncertain) or 'narrative verdict' (a description of the death and circumstances).

METHODS OF SUICIDE

In order to take practical action to minimize the risk of suicide or self-harm, planners need to take account of the ways people choose to end their lives or harm themselves. Over the period 2001–2010, the most common methods in the general population were hanging/strangulation (44%) and self-poisoning/overdose (23%), followed by jumping/multiple injuries (10%, mainly jumping from a height or being struck by a train) (NCI 2013).

In recent years, suicide deaths by hanging increased while those by self-poisoning decreased, as did those by carbon monoxide poisoning, the latter following the introduction of catalytic converters in 1993 (*ibid.*). Suicides by firearms are far less common in the UK than in countries where guns are much more readily available (*ibid.*).

WHO IS AFFECTED?

Across the lifespan

The 2007 Adult Psychiatric Morbidity Survey (NHSIC 2009) found that 17 per cent of people said they had thought about committing suicide at some point in their life, 6 per cent said that they had attempted suicide, and 5 per cent said that they had engaged in self-harm. The rate of each of these broadly declined with age. The proportion of women reporting suicidal thoughts in the past year increased between the 2000 and 2007 surveys. There was also an increase in the proportion of people reporting that they had engaged in self-harm, especially among women aged 16–24.

In the UK in 2011, 75 per cent of the suicides in those aged 15 and over were males. This equates to rates of 18 per 100,000 population in males and 6 per 100,000 population in females (ONS 2013f). (The rates are calculated to take into account the differences in population age and sex structure so that different areas can be compared.)

In 16–24 year-olds, 5 per cent have attempted suicide, compared with 2 per cent of 65–74 year-olds. However, the rate among people more than 85 rises again (RCPsych 2010).

In 2011/2012 in England there were more than 114,000 inpatient admissions for intentional self-harm or an event of undetermined intent (ONS 2013f). In contrast to the trends in completed suicide, the incidence of self-harm has been rising in the UK over the past 20 years. The rate of self-harm is higher in younger people than older people and is more common among women and girls than among men and boys, although completed suicide is more prevalent among men and boys (RCPsych 2010).

Young people

Suicide and injury/poisoning of undetermined intent is the second leading cause of death for 15–19 year-old males (12 per cent of deaths in that group) (ONS 2013f). Children as young as eight have been found to have harmed themselves (RCPsych 2010). However, the rate of self-harm is relatively low in early childhood, increasing rapidly with adolescence, when it often indicates the presence of other problems (NCCMH 2005), some of which will be discussed later in this chapter. The incidence peaks from the ages of 15 to 19 years in females and from 20 to 24 years in males (NCCMH 2012b).

In one survey, the most common reason given by young people (more than 70%) for self-harming was 'escape from a terrible state of mind' (RCPsych 2010). Other reasons include 'death', 'punishment', 'demonstration of desperation', 'wanted to find out if someone loved them', 'attention seeking', 'wanted to frighten someone' and 'wanted to get back at someone'.

Antenatal and post-natal women

Psychiatric disorders, particularly depression, have been found to be the leading cause of maternal deaths in the UK, with more than half of these deaths being a consequence of suicide (NCCMH 2007) and 60 per cent occurring between six weeks before and twelve weeks after delivery.

Adults

Suicide and injury/poisoning of undermined intent is the leading cause of death in England and Wales in both men and women aged 20–34 (accounting for respectively 26 per cent and 13 per cent of deaths in that age group) and in men aged 35–49 (13% of deaths) (ONS 2013d).

Older people

Although older people are less likely to talk about suicide, they are more likely to carry it out (Murphy *et al.* 2012). They are more likely than other groups to have received medical or psychiatric treatment in the previous year (Conwell *et al.* 2010).

Older people are less likely to self-harm but the consequences are often more serious, with perhaps 20 per cent later committing suicide (NCCMH 2004c). There are strong links with self-harm in older people and poor physical health and social isolation (NCCMH 2004c, 2012b). It appears that in older people, unlike the general population, there is little evidence of a link with suicide and socio-economic status but that the overriding factor is depression, with contributory factors of isolation and being divorced or widowed (RCPsych 2010).

Life circumstances

In Chapter 3, we outlined the life circumstances that could contribute to mental ill health. In this subsection we focus largely on factors known to affect suicide risk directly. However, it should be borne in mind also that all of the factors contributing to mental ill health will also contribute to suicide risk because mental ill health (particularly depression) is a risk factor for suicide. The cumulative effect of different factors is also important, and it is likely that suicidal behaviours result from the combination of several factors or circumstances (RCPsych 2010). The order of the topics in this subsection is broadly that of Chapter 3.

Bereavement

People recently bereaved can be very vulnerable and at risk of suicidal behaviour (Church and Ryan n.d.). Particularly vulnerable are those bereaved by suicide, especially mothers and siblings following a child's suicide (RCPsych 2010).

Those who look after people who self-harm are also vulnerable, because of the distress caused by seeing their loved ones self-harming (*ibid.*).

Black and Minority Ethnic groups

There are many inconsistencies among the conclusions of research into the variation in suicide and self-harm between ethnic groups in the UK. Some of the more common findings reported are the following:

- Being white is one of the attributes associated with high risk of suicide (NHSIC 2009).

- South Asian women have been found to be at increased risk of self-harm. 'The reasons identified for this difference include isolation and family pressure from husbands demanding a less Westernized form of behaviour; interference from parents-in-law; arranged marriages or the rejection of an arranged marriage; isolation even within the wider community; cultural conflict; and problems at school, including racist bullying' (RCPsych 2010, p.33). South Asian men have lower rates of self-harm than South Asian women (NCCMH 2012b).

- Women born in Sri Lanka, India and the East African Commonwealth are approximately 50 per cent more likely to die by suicide than the general population as a whole (Church and Ryan n.d.).

- The highest risk for self-harm is in young Black women (NCCMH 2012b).

- An increased risk of suicide has been found in young Caribbean and African men, with some of the difference perhaps as a consequence of variation in access to services (NCCMH 2010b).

- There is some evidence of an increasing risk of self-harm for people of Caribbean origin aged under 35 (RCPsych 2010).

Bullying

Self-harm is sometimes an indicator of a problem such as bullying or domestic violence (NCCMH 2004c). There has in recent months been much publicity about suicides in young people as a result of bullying via social media, as mentioned in Chapter 6.

Carers

Carers and family members of people who self-harm are at risk mainly because they are vulnerable to psychological distress from their caring, particularly if they are parents of young self-harmers or mothers or siblings of young suicides (RCPsych 2010).

Family history

People with a family history of suicide are at greater risk of committing suicide themselves (Church and Ryan n.d.). Similarly, self-harm in family members appears to be a risk factor for self-harm (NCCMH 2012b).

Family structure and relationships

Being divorced is a recognized risk factor for suicide (Church and Ryan n.d.), and self-harm is more common among those who are single or divorced, live alone or are single parents (NCCMH 2012b). Relationship breakdown is frequently a contributory factor for both suicide and self-harm (RCPsych 2010).

Homelessness

As described in Chapter 3, being homeless has significant adverse effects on people's mental health and well-being. Homelessness can be a major contributory factor to suicide (RCPsych 2010).

Unemployment can lead to severe financial problems and to homelessness. Unemployed people, possibly suffering from anxiety and despair, have a much higher risk of suicide than those who are in employment (*ibid.*).

When people are homeless they may also have greater problems accessing the services that may be of help to them so that they may not get preventive treatment, such as counselling.

Offenders

People in prison have very high rates of both self-harm and suicide. Male prisoners are five times more likely than men in the general public to die by suicide, while the rate among young offenders is 18 times higher (RCPsych 2010). Not only sentenced and remand prisoners but also ex-prisoners recently released into the community are at high risk (Church and Ryan n.d.).

It is during the first few months of being in custody that the risk of suicide is highest. It is believed that this is partly because new prisoners are worried about everyday problems such as money and relationships. It can be attributed also to doubts about legal status and also overcrowding in prisons (RCPsych 2010).

Half of female and a quarter of male remand prisoners have been self-harmers, and up to 10 per cent of prisoners may self-harm while in prison, with women's rates more than double the men's. High rates are explained partly because prisoners have high rates of mental illness, past exposure to violence or abuse and drug or alcohol problems (NCCMH 2004c).

Women are affected by additional factors: they are more likely to have young children and they are more likely to be further from home, because there are not so many women's prisons, and are therefore isolated from friends and family (RCPsych 2010).

People with learning disability, long-term conditions or physical disability

Estimates of the extent of self-harm in those with learning disabilities range from below 2 per cent to 24 per cent. Sometimes self-harming behaviour will just be dismissed as challenging behaviour. It is known that self-injury tends to be more serious in those with severe learning disability, and this has been attributed to a 'narrower range of contributing factors than in the general population, including genetically determined syndromes and other physiological factors as well as autism' (RCPsych 2010, p.26). The living conditions of a learning disabled self-harmer may also contribute to self-harm, particularly if there is abuse or neglect, bullying or a feeling of being confined (*ibid.*).

Many chronic physical health problems have been linked to increased risk of suicide, largely because of the depression that can be associated with them (Church and Ryan n.d.). Similarly, many self-harmers had been suffering from a physical health problem at the time of the self-harming (NCCMH 2004c). In children and young people, those with physical disability are at higher risk from mental ill health and behavioural problems, including particularly depression. Because of mood swings in these children, and especially mood swings in adolescents, depression is not always recognized (NCCMH 2005).

Unfortunately, sometimes the prescription drugs used to treat certain conditions can lead to mental health problems, exacerbating any mental problems associated with the condition itself. For example, the anti-obesity drug rimonabant is associated with increasing the chances of depression and suicidal thoughts (NHS Knowledge Services 2007).

People with mental health conditions

In adults, almost two-thirds of suicides occur in people with depression, a rate of suicide more than four times higher than that of the general population. Depression is the leading cause of suicide in older people. Although most common in those with severe depression, there is still an increased risk in those with a less severe condition (NCCMH 2011a).

Several other diagnoses of mental illness have been established as risk factors for completed suicide. About 10 per cent of people with schizophrenia die by suicide (NCCMH 2010b). Death rates in those diagnosed with antisocial personality disorder are higher than those with many other mental health conditions, due in part to suicide and in part to an increase in drug misuse and aggression (Goodwin et al. 2009; NCCMH 2010a). Patients with bipolar disorder are at a higher risk of suicide than the general population (with a rate of 10–15%), particularly during depressed or mixed episodes (NCCMH 2006), and suicide may occur with little warning, especially in those who also have other impulse control disorders such as substance misuse, borderline personality disorder and eating disorder: the rapid switch from mania or hypomania to depression may also be a particular risk for suicide, as may stressful life events.

In children and young people with depression, there is a risk of about 3 per cent of suicide over the next ten years. Certain groups within the young population, such as those with physical or learning disabilities, have higher risks of depression and mental health problems than others. Other groups at risk include young offenders, particularly those in secure institutions, and it is believed that the high rate of suicides there may indicate that serious depression is not being appropriately diagnosed or treated (NCCMH 2005).

Major depression and having certain mental disorders are also risk factors for self-harming behaviour. The group with the highest risk for self-harm is those diagnosed with schizophrenia (NCCMH 2012b). Self-harm is also more common than among the general population in those with bipolar disorder, borderline personality disorder, anxiety disorders, eating disorders and post-traumatic stress disorder (RCPsych 2010). Studies have suggested that high rates are in part as a consequence of depression being inadequately diagnosed or managed (NCCMH 2006).

In the UK, only about a quarter of those who commit suicide have been in contact with mental health services in the year before the suicide (RCPsych 2010). With regard to self-harm, the majority of those who harm themselves do not have a formal psychiatric illness (*ibid.*).

In 2011, there were nearly 1,800 suicides by people receiving mental health services in the UK (two-thirds in males) (NCI 2013). This number has risen partly because of changes in coroners' verdicts and partly because of rising numbers of people diagnosed with problems and therefore under mental health care (*ibid.*). Post-discharge suicides average more than 220 per year and are most common in the first week after leaving hospital. Among those who were inpatients at the time of the suicide, numbers have been falling dramatically. However, on average, 160 suicides per year occur in patients who are under Crisis Resolution/Home Treatment (CR/HT) teams (England, Scotland and Wales). This is more than those who are inpatients and reflects the changes that have taken place in the care of people receiving mental health services.

People suffering shame following arrest or disclosure of offences

There are sometimes high-profile cases of individuals who commit suicide when some aspects of their behaviour, particularly illegal behaviour, become public. Past instances include a popular television and radio celebrity convicted of shoplifting a small cheap item, her first offence. More recently, amid the highly publicized trials related to child sex offences, at least one public official has been reported as committing suicide before his trial began.

Refugees and asylum-seekers

With refugees and asylum-seekers, the adverse circumstances they have been under contribute to their mental ill health, leading to anxiety and depression that, in turn, increase the risk of suicide. Those in prison have even higher rates of both suicide and self-harm than the general prison population (where rates are already much higher than in the general population) (RCPsych 2010).

Sexual or physical abuse, including domestic violence

Childhood abuse, including sexual abuse and domestic violence, is now well recognized as contributing to self-harm and suicidal behaviour (NCCMH 2004c). There are self-harm issues among women, particularly where the abuse was repeated or was sexual abuse by an immediate family member (RCPsych 2010). Where there is a history of childhood sexual abuse, repetition of self-harm is more likely, as is poor general mental health, which in turn contributes to suicide and self-harm risk (NCCMH 2012b).

Sexuality

Evidence of a link between sexual orientation and self-harm has been growing in recent years, with higher risks in the non-heterosexual groups, particularly in young people (NCCMH 2012b). Self-harm in adolescents can be associated with confusion over sexual orientation and sexuality (RCPsych 2010).

A contributory factor is believed to be the increased amounts of bullying and victimization suffered by the lesbian, gay and bisexual populations (NCCMH 2004c). These groups may face prejudice, discrimination, hostility and violence, sometimes in their own families, and their vulnerability to mental health problems may be increased if they are also misusing drugs or alcohol (RCPsych 2010).

Social isolation and inclusion

Self-harm is more common among those who have a severe lack of social support (NCCMH 2012b). Suicide risk is higher in those who are socially isolated, particularly in older people (as mentioned earlier).

Veterans of the armed forces

Young men, aged 24 and younger, leaving the UK military forces, appear to have a risk of suicide with a rate up to three times higher than that of men in that age group in the general population and of men still serving in the forces. It is recognized that many suffer psychological problems following their service career and may have difficulty settling back into civilian life (RCPsych 2010).

Personal behaviours

Personal behaviours affect the likelihood of depression, as outlined in Chapter 4, and depression is a major contributory factor to suicide. Within this subsection, we focus on behaviours that are more specifically linked to committing or being at risk from committing suicide.

Substance misuse

The risk of suicide attempt and death by suicide associated with opioid use disorders and mixed intravenous drug use is greater than that for alcohol misuse (The Scottish Government 2008). Over the past 20 years, UK death rates from acute poisoning with illicit drugs have more than doubled and, in women particularly, there has been a rise in both self-harm and suicide attempts related to drug misuse (RCPsych 2010).

More than 800 suicides a year are in patients who have a history of alcohol misuse (NCI 2013). Studies have shown a consistently high level of alcohol problems among people who kill themselves (Foster 2001). More than half of men presenting at hospital following self-harm have consumed alcohol in the preceding few hours, with half regularly drinking excessively and one-quarter being alcohol dependent (Foster, Gillespie and McLelland 1997). Importantly, it has been shown that reducing alcohol intake leads to reduced likelihood of suicide (Brady 2006).

The risk of suicide from alcohol misuse is greater among women than among men (The Scottish Government 2008). Alcohol consumption is implicated in about half of the incidents of self-harm that result in accident and emergency visits (NCCMH 2012b), and in women there has been an increase in the amount of self-harming behaviour associated with alcohol (RCPsych 2010).

Among people with both bipolar disorder and drug or alcohol problems, the risks of suicide and attempted suicide are increased, partly because the substances misused can adversely affect the illness itself (NCCMH 2006).

Self-harming behaviour and subsequent self-harm or suicide

Of those whose self-harm results in a visit to an emergency department, some 20 per cent will self-harm again within 12 months (NCCMH 2012b).

Whether or not an episode of self-harm was intended to be a suicide, people who self-harm repeatedly are at a high risk of suicide, possibly even 30 times more likely than the general population (RCPsych 2010).

Suicide bombers

As pointed out by the Royal College of Psychiatrists (RCPsych), 'it is impossible to consider the issue of self-harm and suicide in the present international security climate without being aware of so-called "suicide bombers"' (RCPsych 2010, p.35).

Research suggests that 'though religion might play a key role in recruiting potential suicide bombers, the driving force is instead a mixture of motivations, including politics, humiliation, revenge, retaliation and altruism' (Hassan 2009, cited in *ibid.*, p.35). It has also been found that suicide bombers generally do not show signs of mental disorders (*ibid.*).

WIDER DETERMINANTS

The previous section included an outline of personal factors (age and sex, life circumstances and personal behaviours) that appear linked with greater likelihood of suicide. In this section, we consider some of the main external factors that can affect the likelihood of suicide. As mentioned earlier, there are links between suicide and self-harm, so some assessments of risk will have considered both of these together.

As with the subsection on personal behaviours, we focus on issues where there are known links with suicide, rather than just with depression.

Income (employment and unemployment)

Unemployment is linked to an increased risk of suicide (The Scottish Government 2008). Two-thirds of men under the age of 35 with mental health problems who die by suicide are unemployed (Social Exclusion Unit 2004). Rapid and large-scale unemployment has been associated with significant increases in suicide rates (Lundin and Hemmingsson 2009), as has recession (Stuckler, King and McKee 2009). Evidence is emerging of the effects on suicide of the 2008 global financial crisis (HM Government and DH 2012): excess numbers of suicides, linked to unemployment, have occurred in many countries, particularly in men and young people (Hawton and Haw 2013). Being unemployed increases the likelihood of getting into debt, and when people are in debt and/or homeless, they are especially at risk of suicide and self-harm (RCPsych 2010; Social Exclusion Unit 2004).

Of any single occupational group, farmers account for the largest numbers of suicides (Gregoire and Mayers 2006). Certain other occupational groups – unskilled occupations, doctors, nurses and vets – also show increased rates of suicide (Church and Ryan n.d.). It is worth noting that farmers and those in medical-related professions have greater access to the means of suicide (guns in the case of farmers and drugs for the others). Unskilled workers may be among the most deprived of those who are actually in employment, and their risk of depression is heightened, as discussed in Chapter 2.

A stable ecosystem and sustainable resources

As discussed in Chapter 2, environmental factors that improve mental well-being can reduce depression, so reducing the risk of suicide or self-harm.

Historically rates of suicide appear to be lower in rural than urban areas, although the pattern may be changing (Gregoire and Mayers 2006). In Scotland there is a greater risk of suicide in more remote rural areas. A possible reason for increased rates in rural areas is the greater likelihood of social isolation, which can be exacerbated if a mental or physical health condition prevents someone from driving. Access to services has also been raised as an issue: in rural areas it is sometimes more difficult to get to specialist mental health services, so that the beneficial effects of early treatment may be missed. Another important contributory factor is rural poverty – where a rural area is deprived, it will suffer the same problems as any deprived area, but if it sits within a generally wealthy area the problems can be overlooked and can become worse because of being isolated from wider communities or services.

Social justice and equity

Being in the lowest household income quintile has been given as one of the main risk factors of suicide (NHSIC 2009), and self-harm is also more common among people who are socio-economically disadvantaged (NCCMH 2012b).

EFFECTIVE INTERVENTIONS

There is an ever-increasing array of evidence on the effectiveness and cost-effectiveness of treatment or action around suicide and self-harm. Greater cost savings can be made by spending more on the preventive elements, for example by addressing the factors likely to increase suicide, such as depression (JCPMH 2013).

In this section, we focus largely on evidence used in national guidance or guidelines, such as those produced for NICE or the Scottish Intercollegiate Guidelines Network (SIGN), considering it in terms of the five Ottawa Charter areas for action (WHO 1986) discussed earlier (build healthy public policy; strengthen community action; develop personal skills; create supportive environments; and reorientate services).

Build healthy public policy

Policies discussed in Chapter 5 that have a bearing on mental health generally, and depression specifically, are likely to have an impact also on suicide and self-harm, so we do not repeat that material here. Mental health policy, which does refer to suicide, was discussed in Chapter 1, and in Chapter 2 we described how suicides were linked to austerity responses to recession. Although in much of this book we take 'healthy public policy' to mean policy not specifically designed around mental health (or health services), here we mention suicide and self-harm prevention policies. Produced often by departments of health, these are very much multi-agency policies. The suicide prevention strategies of all four nations (DHSS&PS 2011; HM Government and DH 2012; The Scottish Government 2013; Welsh Assembly Government 2009) have broadly similar aims and areas for action, such as: reducing the risk of suicide; helping those affected by it; improving service responses; and improving awareness of the issues. All recognize that action will need to be a coordinated approach across agencies.

Strengthen community action

A wide range of factors increases the risk of suicide and self-harm, many of which are concerned with the local setting or circumstances. In particular, social isolation has a highly significant effect. Social support and connectedness in general is protective against suicide among a range of population groups, including Black Americans and women who have experienced domestic abuse, young adults with severe depression and smokers (The Scottish Government 2008). Consequently, any actions to strengthen contacts within the community, to build social interaction and reduce potential isolation, should help to reduce the risk of suicide and self-harm. National guidance and guidelines tend to stress this aspect, often in relation to specific mental conditions, where the risk is exacerbated. For example:

- For those with bipolar disorder, good-quality social support should be available at times of crisis (NCCMH 2006). Although this may be from just one person, at times a network of social support may be needed. This can be provided through crisis resolution teams, community mental health teams, outpatient services or primary care.

- Adolescents who have attempted suicide are more likely than others to come from neighbourhoods with weak social networks (NCCMH 2005).

- Fostering parental bonding and a healthy family environment could reduce the risk of self-harm in younger people (NCCMH 2012b).

Particular settings may also require the strengthening of social connections. For example, psychosocial interventions should be available to those in prison who have substance abuse problems, with account taken of the time to be served and the individual likelihood of risk (NCCMH 2008).

Activities that promote general mental well-being in the community are an important part of suicide prevention and may rely on any part of the community, such as local community services or local voluntary organizations. The provision of specific venues for activities is an element of community action, along with improvement or maintenance of good outdoor spaces, with all of these aspects contributing particularly to the reduction of social isolation.

The culture in schools, universities, colleges or workplaces can affect the likelihood of suicidal behaviour. Similarly, religious culture can influence this: for example, both Islam and Christianity strongly condemn suicide, so that suicides and suicide attempts are not only upsetting but potentially shameful for believers and their families (RCPsych 2010).

Other issues can also be addressed at a community level. The challenge of reducing stigma, which can seriously affect both mental well-being and the ability to seek help for problems, is a challenge for the community as a whole. In recent years, access to information about mental illness has become easier, particularly with the Internet and the advent of social media. Several well-known figures, such as Stephen Fry (actor, comedian, writer and broadcaster), share very publicly details of mental health problems, helping to dispel the idea that mental illness is something to keep quiet about.

There is, however, also a downside to easy access to material: there are now suicide chatrooms, where people can find out about methods of suicide and discuss their ideas about committing suicide. Social media have also been blamed for a number of suicides, following anonymous but very public bullying. There have been instances of suicide following blackmail, particularly where a young person has sent intimate photographs to an Internet contact (or via sexting – sending pictures by mobile phone), who has threatened to make them public. Authorities and website or social media site managers do take these issues seriously and aim to reduce the possibility of such adverse events. The role of the Internet and the media in general are often cited in policy documents (*ibid.*), since they can be used in a very positive or a very detrimental manner.

Reducing the risk of suicide bombers depends to some extent on communities helping to identify potential risks. Identifying people who may be vulnerable to recruitment into terrorist activity generally is currently being addressed with some energy through the PREVENT component of the UK Government's domestic counterterrorism strategy (HM Government 2010b).

Develop personal skills

Although there may be various coping strategies for people with depression, the picture is less clear for self-harm and for suicide. There is some evidence that problem-solving skills are protective against repetition of self-harm, but it is not certain whether the effect will continue (NCCMH 2012b). Cognitive behavioural therapy has also been found to be effective for those who have self-harmed and, in general, social adjustment skills, participation in sport and engaging with their community are believed to modify the risk of self-harming behaviour (RCPsych 2010).

A number of coping skills requiring an element of self-control including self-efficacy, instrumentality, social adjustment skills, positive future thinking and sublimation appear to be protective against suicidal behaviour, particularly among adolescents and/or at times of stressful life events (The Scottish Government 2008). Being in control of emotions, thoughts and behaviour can mediate against suicide risk associated with sexual abuse among adolescents. There is some evidence that an attitude towards sport as a healthy activity and participation in sporting activity is protective against suicidal behaviour among adolescents (*ibid.*).

Create supportive environments

As well as health and social services (discussed in the next topic), a range of services can contribute to the creation of supportive environments that help to reduce the risk of suicide or self-harm. These will be summarized in a table in the Conclusion, along with services that create supportive environments for the subjects of our other two case studies, young BME groups and those with long-term conditions. Interventions discussed in Chapter 6 will also be of relevance to suicide.

Reducing opportunities for suicide

There are effective, simple measures that can reduce the likelihood of suicide, such as the erection and maintenance of physical barriers to access to high-risk venues such as bridges or cliff-tops. There has been much suicide prevention activity in hospitals, including the removal of weight-bearing curtain rails.

Action by both government and pharmaceutical companies may be needed in connection with the availability of products that provide the means of suicide or self-harm. For example, reducing pack sizes of over-the-counter drugs, such as aspirin and paracetamol, has helped to reduce the severity of outcomes of deliberate overdose.

Reorientate services

The health and social care sectors, as a whole, need to work with other agencies. For example, services in contact with bereaved people can advise on appropriate counselling, perhaps from third-sector organizations such as Cruse. Another example would be services in collaboration with third-sector organizations, erecting signs with contact details for services (such as the Samaritans). Such signs have been found to reduce the numbers of suicides in places such as bridges and cliff-tops.

Liaison with the criminal justice system can also reap benefits. Mental health workers can work with police and prison officers to raise awareness of mental health issues and suicide risk. Within police custody cells or prison, assessments and monitoring of suicide risks can take place. Such assessment or monitoring is also essential for newly released prisoners on probation. Working with the criminal justice system is sometimes just a matter of ensuring good communication, so that people at risk are identified and services are in contact with them. Similarly, communication and good information should be part of the relationship the service has with coroners conducting inquests: some of the coroners' information will come from the health sector, but there will be a need to share information so that lessons learned from any suicide are translated into effective action.

The following subsections consider action or interventions specific to suicide or self-harm that are appropriate to different parts of the health and social care system.

Social services

Examples include the following:

- Where there is direct contact with children, addressing issues such as child abuse and domestic violence, major risk factors for suicide and self-harm, could reduce the risk later in life.
- Because of the extent of the impact of social, family and relationship factors on suicide and self-harm risk, social workers, youth workers and life coaches have a significant role.
- Adult social services can provide day care or respite services, for the benefit of both patients and carers.

(NCCMH 2004c, 2005, 2007, 2010b, 2011a, 2011b)

Primary care and accident and emergency departments

The following are actions that can be taken within primary care and accident and emergency departments (NCCMH 2004c, 2005, 2011c):

- Primary care:
  - Ensure that prescribing practice follows British National Formulary guidelines, and that those at risk, including known drug users, are not given prescriptions for potentially lethal drugs for more than their immediate needs.
  - Rapid assessment of both physical and psychological need, including questions about social support and about thoughts of suicide.
- Accident and emergency departments – pressure to discharge patients from A&E departments means that sometimes people are discharged too soon after an episode of self-harm or a suicide attempt. Appropriate follow-up care or referral is essential. It is also important that staff act in a non-judgemental manner.

Secondary care hospital-based services in mental health

Recommendations for services from the National Confidential Inquiry into Suicide and Homicide by People with Mental Illness (NCI 2013) stress the need for a holistic approach to patient care. Examples include a recommendation to address the economic difficulties of patients who may be at risk of suicide, ensuring they receive advice on debts, housing and employment. Patients with mental health problems should also undergo physical health checks, and their use of prescription medicines needs to be monitored.

In line with this holistic approach, the NCCMH refers to the need for person-centred care, taking into account service users' needs and preferences, paying attention to physical and environmental needs and supporting patients to manage factors that have contributed to their mental health crisis. Continuity of care and smooth transitions are also recommended (NCCMH 2011c).

Alcohol and drugs services

Key recommendations (NCI 2013) include the maintenance of services for dual diagnosis and being vigilant about the suicide risk from opiates. The NCI also recommends a strengthening of specialist services and risk management for patients who are misusing alcohol and drugs.

Community-based mental health services

Many mental health conditions can be treated in the community, rather than in a hospital setting. NHS mental health services make use of teams of staff working outside the hospital and, in general, there is an aim of only admitting patients when absolutely necessary (for example, when there is suicidal behaviour).

NHS treatment in the community may be intensive, such as that provided by assertive outreach teams or home-based treatment. It frequently takes the form of counselling and provision of supportive relationships. The support is essential particularly for lifelong or long-term conditions or disorders, such as antisocial personality disorder (NCCMH 2010a).

The Samaritans is one third-sector organization with particular focus on potential suicide. Papyrus is a national UK charity dedicated to the prevention of suicide in young people. Many other third-sector organizations provide advice, self-help groups, counselling or practical help for those with mental health problems and their families or carers. Third-sector organizations also undertake research and campaigns, raise awareness, moderate websites and provide staff training. Statutory organizations can contract with third-sector organizations to provide expert services.

For those self-harmers who have not been in contact with mental health services (the majority), third-sector organizations may be a more acceptable way of finding help because of stigma and the difficulties of navigating around the health system (RCPsych 2010).

User and carer involvement

As with other groups of people, it is essential that those who self-harm or attempt suicide are involved in the development of suicide prevention strategies and in decisions about their own care or treatment. Families and carers may also need to be involved. Recognizing that the relationships service users have with their families may not always be helpful, the Royal College of Psychiatrists suggests that:

> [p]rofessionals should regard it as automatic to enquire about the service user's carer and the level of involvement that they would like to see from them. If there is a joint agreement that the carer be involved, they should be kept informed on situations that concern them, especially when it directly relates to their care giving. (RCPsych 2010, p.70)

After a suicide, consistent support for immediate family members and close friends or carers is important, with referral to specialist services if appropriate, although the rarity of the event may make this difficult for generic services.

Integrated care

The need for and the benefits of integrated care have been discussed in Chapters 5 and 6. With regard to suicide and self-harm, all the organizations involved are expected to work together not only with individual patients but also in drawing up any suicide prevention plans.

Measuring quality and equity

There has already been reference to the need for services to provide equal and fair services to all patients, with specific mention of groups such as those who self-harm (to be treated with the same respect as other patients); patients from BME groups (to be treated in a culturally appropriate way); and young people (to be admitted to age-appropriate facilities).

Patient Recorded Experience Measures and Patient Recorded Outcome Measures were discussed in Chapter 1, along with Clinician

Recorded Outcome Measures. All of these can contribute to an evaluation of services.

Audits of quality and equity are recommended by the National Suicide Prevention Strategy Advisory Group (Church and Ryan n.d.). There are different types of audit. A 'suicide audit' looks at records of suicides and provides information on such things as the victims, their situations, methods of suicide and contacts with services. Suicides can also be reviewed using techniques such as Significant Event Analysis or Root Cause Analysis, which help to identify points along the pathway to suicide where improvements could be made that may prevent the suicide. A 'clinical audit' compares actual practice to standards and helps to identify potentially beneficial changes in practice. The Advisory Group identified the need to record more detailed information on suicide following deliberate self-harm and on suicides from different ethnic minority groups and different occupations. This type of information can be used in an assessment of fairness or equity of the delivery of services and to identify any gaps in service. Frequently considered alongside suicide audits are drug-related death reviews, analysing the factors surrounding deaths associated with drugs, regardless of whether the death was intended.

When Wales's national suicide and self-harm action plan was developed (Welsh Assembly Government 2009), it was based on an overall population approach but wanted to ensure that there was a focus on particular groups known to be at raised risk and on tackling health and social inequalities. An equality Impact Assessment was carried out to consider this. The particular groups of people known to be at particular risk of exclusion, inequity and suicide included: young people; older people; socially excluded homeless people; people who are gay, lesbian, bisexual or transgendered; offenders; people from minority ethnic groups; and people with a mental illness. Significant risk factors for communities and the people living within them are unemployment, poverty, social isolation and deprivation. A consultation process around the equality audit led to changes in emphasis in the policy to ensure that there was adequate focus on those at highly increased risk of suicide and self-harm.

PRINCIPLES INTO PRACTICE

This extended case study was chosen as an example of a very specific and relatively rare event, which requires a broad-based public health approach across disciplines and agencies for a concern with prevention and reduction of harm. Suicide in some ways seems the ultimate personal choice. Yet this chapter has shown that even here the social, cultural, political and environmental context plays a crucial role, in line with our second principle that we must address these 'determinants of health' if we are to enhance mental health and well-being. The analysis around lifespan, life circumstances, personal behaviour and wider determinants to this issue helps demonstrate how the application of our third principle – the assessment of health care need in the population concerned and the use of systematically assessed evidence about what works – can benefit service planners. We hope it is also helpful for those on the front line to see their role in any part of the system in context. Finally, our fourth principle, involving communities, users and carers in framing priorities, has also been applied in this extremely sensitive area of work.

Chapter 8

EXTENDED CASE STUDY

IMPROVING MENTAL HEALTH AND WELL-BEING AMONG YOUNG BLACK AND MINORITY ETHNIC GROUPS

KEY POINTS

- BME groups are diverse: South Asian women are particularly at risk of mental health disorders.

- Many BME groups experience endemic racism and discrimination, but live in strongly cohesive communities: addressing these issues requires strong community involvement.

- BME populations tend to be over-represented in the social housing sector, and have high levels of homelessness.

- BME children are over-represented among looked-after children, whereas Asian children are under-represented.

- BME young carers particularly experience isolation, having little support or opportunities for leisure and socializing, and there are high levels of bereavement.

- BME women experience higher rates of domestic violence and sexual abuse, including female genital mutilation (FGM).

- Young BME LGBT populations face more homophobia than their peers.

- Unhealthy personal behaviours involving tobacco, drugs and alcohol may be used as coping mechanisms, and sexual health is poor among young BME groups.

- Poverty and unemployment affect far higher proportions of BME young people than white.
- BME young people have very different experiences of crime when compared with the white population, both as victims and as suspects or perpetrators.

INTRODUCTION

In this chapter, we consider mental health issues for young Black and Minority Ethnic (BME) groups. Those groups are affected both by problems specific to all ages of people in BME groups and by any issues affecting young people of any ethnicity (including, for example, the fertility rate and the health or treatment of antenatal and post-natal women).

There is no standard definition for the term 'young'. Some health or social services may cater for young people up to the age of 16, others 18 and sometimes it can be taken to be 25.

The Department of Health in England takes BME groups to mean:

All people of minority ethnic status in England. It does not only refer to skin colour but to people of all groups who might experience discrimination and disadvantage, such as those of Irish origin, those of Mediterranean origin and East European migrants. (DH 2005, p.11)

In England and Wales, approximately 14 per cent of the population are classified as 'non-white': 2.5 per cent are Indian, 2.2 per cent mixed, 2.0 per cent Pakistani, 0.8 per cent Bangladeshi, 0.7 per cent Chinese, 1.5 per cent other Asian, 1.8 per cent African, 1.1 per cent Caribbean, 0.5 per cent other black and 1 per cent other ethnic groups (ONS 2013a). There are other minority groups (for example, Jews) that are not classified under the census definitions as ethnic minorities but can experience cultural and mental health issues in the same way as ethnic minorities.

As with the other two case studies, the sequence of headings from Chapter 2 ('Wider determinants'), Chapter 3 ('Life circumstances') and Chapter 4 ('Personal behaviours') is used wherever relevant. Because it is focusing on young people, the headings from 'Across the lifespan' are not relevant. The final part of the study uses the headings from Chapters 5 and 6 to discuss effective interventions.

WHO IS AFFECTED?

After age is taken into account, the Adult Psychiatric Morbidity Survey found little variation between white, Black and South Asian men in England in the rates of any common mental disorder (anxiety or depression); however, in women all common mental disorders (except phobias) were more prevalent in the South Asian group (NHSIC 2009).

Some issues for people with mental health problems are even worse for people in ethnic minority groups (Social Exclusion Unit 2004). They include stigma and discrimination (with the added burden of racial discrimination) and social exclusion (with mental health problems exacerbating the exclusion issues that ethnic minority populations already experience). It is recognized that poverty can also help to explain some of the differences (Mental Health Foundation n.d. a), as BME groups can be among the most deprived groups in the population.

Several reports (e.g. Bansal *et al.* 2014; Francis and Smith 2002; NIMHE 2005) have shown that, with regard to mental health services, BME groups are more likely to experience:

- problems in accessing services, particularly talking treatments
- lower satisfaction with services
- cultural and language barriers in assessments
- lower GP involvement in care and inadequate community-based crisis care
- lower involvement of service users, family and carers
- an adverse pathway into mental health services:
  - ∘ higher compulsory admission rates to hospital
  - ∘ higher involvement in legal system and forensic settings
  - ∘ higher rates of transfer to medium- and high-secure facilities
- higher voluntary admission rates to hospital
- lower effectiveness of hospital treatment, longer hospital stays and higher readmission rates

- less likelihood of having social care/psychological needs addressed within care planning/treatment processes
- more severe and coercive treatments.

Some of these differences may be 'because mainstream mental health services often fail to understand or provide services that are acceptable and accessible to non-white British communities and meet their particular cultural and other needs' (Mental Health Foundation n.d. a). Some minority groups may be reluctant to engage with health services and there may also be some over-diagnosis of mental health problems in people whose first language is not English (*ibid.*).

There is, of course, great diversity within BME groups, in health profiles, lifestyle and life circumstances. Issues associated with different ethnic groups vary:

- Irish people living in the UK have higher hospital admissions for mental health problems than the general UK population, with particularly high rates of depression, alcohol-related problems and suicide.
- African-Caribbean people have low rates of common mental disorders but higher diagnosed rates of schizophrenia and are more likely to be treated under a section of the Mental Health Act 1983 (England and Wales).
- Statistics on Asian people with mental health problems are inconsistent, but this group seems to have better rates of recovery from schizophrenia, low suicide rates in men and older people and higher suicide rates in young women. There are high rates of alcohol problems among Indian men.
- There is little knowledge of the extent of mental health problems in the Chinese community. (*ibid.*)

In terms of recovery from mental ill health in BME communities, Seebohm (2008) identifies the importance of: paid user involvement, which can aid service change; personal and health development opportunities, particularly in the arts; access to education, training, and paid and voluntary employment; group activities, including self-help; and promoting positive role models.

Life circumstances

The order of topics in this subsection again mirrors that of Chapter 3 as far as possible.

Arranged and forced marriage

Marriages arranged by a third party rather than the two participants are common in many countries, often seen as a positive way of making a suitable match (Sardar 2008). However, arranged marriages can entail early and forced marriage: across the world, approximately 14 million marriages take place with the female being under 18 years of age. Although under 16 year-olds cannot legally get married in the UK, families, particularly those from South East Asia and parts of Africa, send girls away from the UK to enter into early, arranged and sometimes forced marriage (Plan n.d.). The impact on girls is immediate and long term, with increased chances of them leaving education, being more likely to live in poverty, experience high levels of sexual violence, and having poor sexual, reproductive and maternal health, including increased rates of human immunodeficiency virus (HIV)/acquired immunodeficiency syndrome (AIDS) and high infant mortality (United Nations Population Fund 2012).

Bereavement

Young BME groups are more likely to experience early bereavement, given that there is a greater proportion of this group growing up in more deprived circumstances, and this in itself is related to higher mortality rates (Fauth, Thompson and Penny 2009). Access to specialist mental health services is limited, as a consequence of barriers relating to discrimination and racism, family and community pressures and the stigma around mental health problems. Within services, a lack of targeting and cultural competence has been shown to be an issue (Kurtz and Street 2006).

Bullying

Identifying bullying within a racist context is complicated. Martin and Hart (2011) found that young people make strong links between poverty and being bullied, often associated with how they look, and particularly how they dress. Young people from ethnic minorities are more likely to come from deprived backgrounds, so are more at risk of bullying. However, most research shows that young people who are members of a BME group are more likely to be a victim of bullying than their white peers. In some areas, high levels of racial bullying have been associated with high rates of ethnic victimization in the local community. Verbal abuse, with name calling about race and colour, is the most common form of bullying, with mixed research findings about the incidence of physical bullying (Butler 2007).

Carers

Approximately 30 per cent of children who are carers in the UK support parents with mental health problems, and more than 15 per cent of them are from BME backgrounds (SCIE 2005). Young BME carers have a range of activities, from household chores, to helping with personal and medical care, as well as interpreting (Jones, Jeyasingham and Rajasooriya 2002). Some of these responsibilities had an impact on their health, well-being and education, and none of the families or young people received adequate or appropriate support, and some even experienced discrimination (*ibid.*). A Barnardo's study (Mills 2003) also found that young Black carers particularly experienced isolation, having little support or opportunities for leisure and socializing.

Family structure and relationships

To the extent that family structure and household composition can be generalized, BME populations tend to have a higher birth rate than the indigenous population of the UK, although this is mainly found in Pakistani, Bangladeshi and mixed-race groups (Phoenix and Husain 2007).

An ONS study (Penn and Lambert 2002) found a large difference between ethnic groups as to ideal family size, with Indian and Pakistani respondents favouring significantly larger families. Both Christians and Muslims showed a preference for larger families than those with no religion. Attitudes to ideal family size closely relate to actual patterns of fertility (*ibid.*).

BME households are conventionally made up of extended families, particularly those from South Asia. Black families, particularly from Caribbean backgrounds, are often seen as having absent fathers, although that does not mean that the father does not participate in supporting the family (Greene, Pugh and Roberts 2008).

Social barriers are particularly relevant to BME parents. For Asian mothers, isolation can be a particular problem, exacerbated by being distanced from their own families, living with their partner's family and having poor English language skills. Many parenting support programmes originate from a white middle-class value system, which may not recognize different cultural attitudes to raising a family (Katz, La Placa and Hunter 2007).

For all families, kin networks are important, but the ways in which they are manifested is coloured by the culture in which they are embedded. This can lead to judgemental attitudes, such as white professionals considering that Black families discipline their children too harshly, whereas Black and Asian parents think white parents lack commitment to parenting, so that children are lacking in respect and undisciplined (Phoenix and Husain 2007).

Homelessness

Nationally, BME communities experience a disproportionate amount of homelessness when compared to the total population, with BME households being three times more likely to experience homelessness than their white counterparts (Steele and Ahmed 2007).

Various reasons have been proposed for these high levels of homelessness, with four main factors identified (Beider and Netto 2012):

- changing household composition, caused by family conflict, domestic abuse, breakdown and overcrowding
- problems with finances
- poor options around housing
- wider policy issues affecting gender-based violence, asylum-seekers and refugees.

Looked-after children

Black and mixed-race children are over-represented among looked-after children, whereas Asian children are under-represented. Black Caribbean children are almost twice as likely as Bangladeshi children to be placed in residential care. Pakistani, Indian and Bangladeshi children are more likely to be returned to their parents than Chinese, Black African or Black Caribbean children.

Factors involved in these differing rates seem to relate to lack of access to appropriate services, under-reporting of concerns in some cultures, and uncertainty on the behalf of services to respond appropriately to the needs of ethnic minority families (Owen and Stratham 2009). BME children entering the adoption and fostering arena are less likely to have core assessments completed and are less likely to be adopted or fostered. Suitable BME adopters have more choice of children, because there are smaller numbers (Thomas 2013).

Offenders

Black offenders tend to be over-represented in the criminal justice system, whereas Asians are under-represented when compared to their white counterparts. Offences are most likely to be violence against the person, handling stolen goods and theft. Black and mixed-race males are more likely to receive a custodial sentence than white men. In contrast, Asian females are less likely to receive a custodial sentence than white women, although their offences tend to be less serious.

Most offenders have been excluded from school at some point, and this was more likely if they were of mixed race (May, Gyateng and Bateman 2009). In *Improving Health, Supporting Justice* (DH 2009a), the national delivery plan of the Health and Criminal Justice Programme Board, it was identified that more than 70 per cent of prisoners suffer from two or more mental disorders.

People with learning disability, long-term conditions or physical disability

There is a paucity of research into the prevalence and needs of BME young people with disabilities (Stalker and Moscardini 2012). Young BME people with learning disabilities are under-represented when it comes to access to services, and may face further isolation because of exclusion from education and employment (Raghavan and Pawson 2009). Depression is recognized as being one of the commonest causes of distress among people with learning disabilities. However, there is mixed evidence around the impact race has on this group (Daniels 2012). The OCC School Exclusions Inquiry found that a Black Caribbean boy who has special educational needs (SEN), and is also from a low-income household, is 168 times more likely to be excluded permanently from school than their white female classmate who is from a more affluent background and does not have SEN (Davis 2012).

People with mental health conditions

The ONS (Hicks 2013) recently used the Annual Population Survey 2011–2012 to ask people to assess their own well-being (see also Chapter 1). People from Black ethnic groups were least satisfied with their lives (6.7 out of 10), compared to Bangladeshi (7 out of 10) and white (7.4 out of 10). All ethnic groups gave lower ratings than whites when asked if they felt the things they do are worthwhile. They also reported higher levels of anxiety. The study recognized that some differences may be as a consequence of the way the questions were worded, as well as the importance of the wider determinants of good mental health.

BME populations are more at risk of experiencing poverty, homelessness, unemployment and other factors associated with poor mental health (Marmot 2010b). Racism itself affects mental health (King *et al.* 2009). Many people from ethnic minority backgrounds fear mental health issues, as they can be stigmatized in their communities, and admission of such a problem may lead to ostracism within their social and family networks. Such fears can lead to a lack of knowledge of services and reluctance to ask for help, which is compounded by mental health services not being sensitive to need (Seebohm *et al.* 2005).

All ethnic groups experience mental health issues in different ways, with differences between groups and from the dominant white population (Greene *et al.* 2008). Young Black men are six times more likely to be sectioned under the Mental Health Act 1983 for compulsory treatment than their white counterparts (BME Leadership Forum 2013). There are complex reasons for this, but it is likely that this is a result of, or is exacerbated by, the oppression and social injustice that this group experiences (Keating *et al.* 2002).

Children and young people of BME parents with a mental health problem may be more vulnerable to a range of poor experiences and outcomes, including bullying, raised stress levels, greater likelihood of mental health problems, greater risk of being taken into care, and failing to complete education because of caring responsibilities (Greene *et al.* 2008).

Refugees and asylum-seekers

In 2011, the United Nations High Commissioner for Refugees (2012) found that 34 per cent of asylum-seekers worldwide were under 18 years old. The experience of refugees and asylum-seekers is varied and may be extremely traumatic, including having lived through war and persecution. Dealing with the aftermath of loss, disruption and sometimes terror, compounded by the complex legal immigration processes, as well as language, cultural and social differences, can have a serious impact on the health of these groups (Sleijpen, ter Heide and Kleber 2013).

The perception of discrimination can lead young refugees to experience mental health and social adaptation problems (Montgomery and Foldspang 2008). The reviewed literature shows that children and young people generally underutilize mental health services, and this is much more likely to be the case with those who are refugees (De Anstiss et al. 2009).

One study in Newcastle (Regional Youth Work Unit and Save the Children 2003) found that young BME asylum-seekers and refugees were particularly isolated and did not access services easily. There were few workers available who were from a similar background, and professionals did not have enough information about the issues for these groups.

Sexual or physical abuse

Black women experiencing physical or sexual abuse are consistently at risk of depression, anxiety, nightmares, pain, post-traumatic stress disorder, substance abuse and a raft of other symptoms (Lacey et al. 2013).

BME women experience higher rates of domestic violence, and because of their underprivileged social circumstances are likely to have poorer outcomes (Allen 2012; Lacey et al. 2013). They are likely to hide domestic abuse in order to preserve family honour and are less likely to divulge information to professionals, because of a fear of lack of confidentiality and gossiping within the community (Wellock 2010).

Children and young people from BME backgrounds, as well as refugees, are at increased risk of abuse from extended family members and of forced marriage, particularly if the young person is lesbian, gay, bisexual or transgender (Jones 2011).

Female genital mutilation (FGM) is a cultural ritual among ethnic groups in 27 countries in sub-Saharan and Northeast Africa, and to a lesser extent in Asia and the Middle East (UNICEF 2013). It involves the total or partial removal of the external sexual organs or any other injury to the female genitals for non-medical reasons (WHO 2010). Nearly 100,000 girls in England and Wales were thought to be at risk of FGM in 2007 (Dorkenoo, Morison and Macfarlane 2007). It has been described as 'a cruel act perpetrated by parents and extended family members upon young girls who are entrusted to their care' (RCM *et al.* 2013, p.6).

The majority of women who have undergone genital mutilation suffer from chronic mental and psychosocial problems, with one in six suffering from post-traumatic stress disorder and one-third suffering from depression or anxiety (Vloeberghs *et al.* 2012). There can also be feelings of fear, nightmares and a higher risk of psychosomatic diseases (Utz-Billing and Kentenich 2008). In addition, feelings of shame and betrayal can develop when the women move outside their traditional circles and learn that their condition is not the norm (Abdulcadira *et al.* 2011).

Sexuality

BME lesbian, gay and bisexual (LGB) communities experience a range of issues that differ from white LGB communities (DH 2007a):

- They are disproportionately affected by homophobic harassment, abuse and violence.
- They are less likely to consider suicide, possibly explained by strong religious and cultural taboos in BME communities. This is not the case for South Asian women, who are more at risk of attempted suicide and self-harm.
- They are more likely to encounter racism and heterosexism when accessing health services.
- They are more likely to maintain contact with BME heterosexual social networks.
- Young BME LGB people are less involved in gay social activities.

Social isolation and inclusion

The background of many ethnic minority groups of living in the UK is a continuing experience of racial discrimination, with the majority of

British people believing that the number of immigrants coming into the UK should be reduced (DCLG 2011a). This finding has been consistent for several years. Attitudes are influenced by a range of factors, although the most significant is level of education (*ibid.*).

Many of the factors that lead to social isolation and those that help to improve inclusion were identified in Chapter 3 and Chapter 6. Within ethnic minority communities, social networks can be critical in maintaining relationships and reducing isolation (McCabe *et al.* 2013). Garner and Bhattacharyya (2011) identify an ongoing debate around ethnicity as to whether minority groups 'self-segregate', and so choose not to integrate. Local segregation can be a double-edged sword: strong local social bonds provide security and support, but can provide a disincentive to move into other areas with higher employment opportunities (Batty *et al.* 2010).

Persistent segregation of BME communities in deprived areas of the UK has been identified as both a symptom and cause of ethnic inequalities, and indicates the lack of integration of ethnic groups into the wider society (Phillips and Harrison 2010). However, promoting policies that increase the ethnic mix of communities, as governments have aimed to do, can lead to weakened social networks, which can be critical in maintaining good mental health, and not be sensitive to the specific needs of minority households (Harries and Richardson 2009).

Members of ethnic minorities are more likely than white people to say they are influential in local decision making, including campaigning and involvement in community organizations (DCLG 2011a). Voting can be considered an indicator of engagement in the society in which a person lives (Hothi *et al.* 2008). Ethnic minorities are as likely to vote as the white British, but are somewhat less likely to be registered. This may be a consequence of both lack of knowledge about eligibility and language barriers. BME people are highly supportive of the Labour party, with two-thirds voting this way; this does not appear to be linked to social class in the way it is in the white population (Heath and Khan 2012). However, it remains the case that Black, ethnic and religious minorities are under-represented in Parliament (DCLG 2011a).

Veterans of the armed forces

Since the Second World War, recruitment from the BME groups has risen as the ethnic mix in the UK has changed. BME men and women make up 5.6 per cent of the Armed Forces, which means that they are still under-represented, although the figure is higher among the younger population (Howarth 2011).

Personal behaviours
Healthy eating

The prevalence of obesity varies across ethnic groups for all age groups, with different groups having different physiological mechanisms for fat storage and having considerably different diets. Generally, Black African women have the highest rates of obesity when using waist circumference, whereas Bangladeshi women do when waist-to-hip ratios are used. Chinese men and women have the lowest levels of obesity, regardless of the measure used. The National Child Measurement Programme shows that obesity in Bangladeshi boys appears to be increasing (NOO 2011). It should also be borne in mind that cultural attitudes to weight may vary.

An extensive American survey found that young Black people had higher dietary fats than young white people, and were more likely to be overweight (Winkelby *et al.* 1999). Men from most ethnic groups, however, have been found to be more likely to consume five or more portions of fruit and vegetable per day than white men (Higgins and Dale 2010).

Physical activity

Young Black people are less likely to be physically active than their white peers (Winkelby *et al.* 1999). South Asian and Chinese women are less likely to meet physical activity guidelines than white women, as were Pakistani and Bangladeshi men. Education was found to be an important predictor of exercise levels (Higgins and Dale 2010).

Alcohol

Most BME groups have higher rates of abstinence, with those from South Asian backgrounds being most likely to drink no alcohol, although those that do drink do so more heavily than other non-white groups. Alcohol consumption has changed and varies by generation: frequent and heavy drinking has increased for Chinese men and Indian women; the proportion of Sikh girls drinking has increased, while second-generation Sikh men are less likely to drink (Hurcombe, Bayley and Goodman 2010).

One study found that those who experience the greatest levels of racial discrimination were likely to drink more alcohol and smoke more, suggesting that unhealthy personal behaviours are used as coping mechanisms (Borrell *et al.* 2010). This is confirmed by the finding that those who live in areas that are more densely populated with similar ethnic groups tend to drink less alcohol (Becares, Nazroo and Stafford 2011).

Smoking

In the 1970s, smoking was much less prevalent in ethnic minorities than the national prevalence. By 1992, this had changed considerably, with Black Caribbeans being as likely to smoke as the white population. By 2004, smoking prevalence was lower in Indians, but higher in Pakistani and considerably higher in Bangladeshi men (Whitrow, Harding and Maynard 2010). There are clear gender differences, with South Asian women being least likely to smoke. Ethnic minorities start smoking at about the same age as their white peers (HEA 1999).

Illicit drug use

Illicit drug use varies across ethnic groups, with those from mixed backgrounds being more likely to have taken any drug in the last year. Asians have the lowest levels of illicit drug use. Black or Black British groups are less likely than white or mixed groups to have taken illegal drugs, although Black Caribbeans have high use of cannabis and so have the highest rates of drug use. However, white and mixed-ethnic groups have the highest use of Class A drugs (Hoare and Moon 2010).

Sexual health

In the UK, young people from BME communities 'continue to be disproportionately affected by poor sexual health' (Mironski 2010, p.5). There are many reasons for this, such as patterns of travel and migration, diverse sexual behaviours and attitudes, and access to appropriate services. A further key element is the strong link between sexually transmitted infections and social deprivation (McDaid, Ross and Young 2012).

In 2011, 49 per cent of Black women had a repeat abortion, compared to 36 per cent of white women (DH 2013a).

There are differing rates of sexually transmitted infections, for example gonorrhoea and chlamydia, among different ethnic groups (Low, Sterne and Barlow 2001). The Health Protection Agency (2012) identified that the rates of gonorrhoea in the 'Black Other' group were 15 times higher than the white British rate, whereas the rate for Indians was about half the white British rate.

Diagnosis of HIV is greater in BME populations, with a 46 per cent higher heterosexual diagnosis rate of Black Africans compared to whites (The UK Collaborative Group for HIV and STI Surveillance 2006). In London in 2011, more than a third of people accessing HIV care were Black African (Forde and Crook 2013).

WIDER DETERMINANTS

Shelter

BME populations tend to be over-represented in the social housing sector, although there are considerable differences between groups, with some less likely to be housed in this sector. Black, Bangladeshi and mixed-heritage households are concentrated in social housing, whereas Indian and Pakistani groups have high rates of home ownership in comparison (Markkanen et al. 2008). Black households are more than twice as likely to live in social housing as others, regardless of the area they live in. Indian households are only 50 per cent as likely as others to live in social housing – again, regardless of where they live (Ferguson et al. 2008).

Ethnic diversity tends to increase in areas of social housing, as most vacancies are a consequence of the death of tenants, who tend to be older and white, and new tenancies are sought by young BME people, who have often recently come to live in the UK (ibid.). One of the reasons BME groups live in particular areas is the strong social networks that they have, which has a considerable influence on their housing decisions (Beider 2012).

The need for social housing is affected by poverty. Given that ethnic populations are more likely to live in poverty (Barnard and Turner 2011), it is unsurprising that they make up a higher proportion of those households living in social housing. The family composition can have an impact on the type of housing needs, with lone parents and larger families being more common within BME populations (Markkanen *et al.* 2008).

Housing policy plays a key role in how people live within the UK. Issues about what policy should be addressing and how it should be addressing it have been debated for many decades. In terms of the ethnic population, perhaps the most critical one has been about how to achieve community cohesion and whether promoting mixed neighbourhoods is the most appropriate way to achieve this (Flint 2010), as mentioned under 'Social isolation and inclusion' above.

Education

The three characteristics that mostly affect educational attainment are ethnicity, socio-economic status and gender (Barnard and Turner 2011). Qualifications and skills are increasingly being found to be of critical importance in addressing child poverty (Bradshaw *et al.* 2006). In turn, childhood poverty is associated with poor educational attainment, leading to poverty (Smith and Middleton 2007), which emphasizes the importance of understanding the relationship between poverty, education and ethnicity.

Tackey, Barnes and Khambhaita (2011) summarize research about the differential impact of education on ethnic groups at each stage of the educational journey. During the early years, some ethnic minority groups, including Black Caribbean, Black African and those with English for Speakers of Other Languages (ESOL) needs, make better progress than white British children. At primary school level, children of mixed white and Asian heritage do best, while mixed white and Black Caribbean children do less well than average. By secondary school, poverty is the largest driver of differential performance, but there are also notable gender disparities, with boys (especially Black Caribbean boys and white boys from deprived households) doing worse. Post-16 Pakistani and Bangladeshi young people achieve fewest qualifications. Post-18 students from ethnic minority groups are less likely to achieve a higher degree class.

BME children and young people tend to achieve higher levels of educational attainment than their white counterparts from similar backgrounds. Social class has a greater impact on white British pupils than on other ethnic groups (Strand 2008), and within lower socio-economic groups, Chinese and Indian pupils make progress at a faster rate than any other groups (Strand 1999). However, Barnard and Turner (2011) identify serious concerns about the treatment and performance of Black Caribbean and Traveller children.

Overall, some groups overcome the evident disadvantage of ethnicity in the early stages of education, and participation in education for post-16 year-olds is high in many ethnic minority groups. There is limited research on the reasons for this, but it has generally been attributed to the largely positive cultural attitudes of ethnic groups to education in general, and in higher education particularly (Tackey *et al.* 2011).

Income (employment and unemployment)

Black and ethnic groups are much more likely to live in poverty than white British people, throughout the UK (Institute of Race Relations n.d.). This is reflected in the poor employment rates of people from differing ethnic backgrounds: in June 2012, 7.3 per cent of white British people were unemployed, compared to 15.5 per cent of Black people and 17.3 per cent of people with mixed ethnicity (*ibid.*). These differences become more stark when unemployment figures for young people are examined, with 26 per cent of Black males aged 16–24 being out of work compared with 16 per cent of their counterparts who are Asian or white (*ibid.*).

Asian populations tend to have different employment status according to gender, with only one in four Pakistani and Bangladeshi women in employment, with almost half looking after the family or home, compared to 20 per cent or fewer in other groups. Tackey *et al.* (2006) found that women from these backgrounds who did want to work were motivated by a desire to free themselves from their traditional roles of financial dependence on their husbands. A shift in attitudes is leading to Bangladeshi women having a more positive view of working outside the home, and this is particularly enhanced where they have female role models in work. The most significant barrier relates to caring responsibilities, particularly childcare, which is exacerbated by having large families (Yeandle *et al.* 2006).

Muslim groups report the highest level of discrimination in employment when compared to other religious groups, although

Sikhs and Hindus also report unfair treatment. Discrimination on the grounds of religion appears to override that of skin colour, with white Muslims experiencing disadvantage in employment over white non-Muslims (Woodhead 2009). Bangladeshi and Pakistani men are more likely to have stopped working in their 40s and 50s, the time when most working-age people in Britain are at the height of their productive capacity. This has been found to be mainly a consequence of ill health (Tackey *et al.* 2006). Overall, Bangladeshi and Pakistani people tend to have low levels of education and qualifications, as well as limited experience, fewer networks in other sectors of the population and low levels of confidence (*ibid.*).

Afro-Caribbean and African men have the highest average risk of unemployment, but this varies within the group according to a range of individual characteristics, with those who have low education levels, live in a disadvantaged area and live alone being at particular risk of unemployment (Berthoud 1999).

A further group that is disadvantaged in the employment market comprises refugees and asylum-seekers. A lack of cultural knowledge has been identified as a key barrier to employment, as well as a lack of social capital (Booker and Boice 2007).

Migrant workers, many of whom come to the UK with high levels of skills and qualifications, often have to take jobs on low wages, as a consequence of employers not recognizing credentials. They are at particular risk of exploitation, especially when newly arrived (Low Pay Commission 2013). At even greater risk are illegal workers. It is estimated that there are more than 600,000 illegal immigrants in the UK. Their opportunities for employment are limited and, if a job is procured, working conditions are likely to be exploitative (Sigona and Hughes 2012). Furthermore, not all illegal immigrants have come to the UK by choice and may be trafficked workers, brought into the country to provide forced labour, including sex work and slavery (National Crime Agency n.d.).

Because ethnic minority groups in employment are more likely to be on a low wage, they are likely to experience difficulties in paying for food, rent, fuel and transport. This group has the added barriers of unequal access to opportunities for career development, stigma and discrimination, as well as not having their skills and experience recognized or valued (Hudson *et al.* 2013).

The concentration of some ethnic minorities in certain areas, such as Pakistanis in West Yorkshire and the North West of England, has an impact on employment opportunities, given the decline in industry in northern England's industrial cities (Yeandle *et al.* 2006).

A stable ecosystem and sustainable resources
Environment

Across the UK, there are areas of high concentrations of some ethnic minority populations. London is the most ethnically diverse city. There are significant differences as to where particular ethnic groups live, with 80 per cent of Black Africans living in London and 80 per cent of Pakistanis living in the Midlands, West Yorkshire and England's north-western towns and cities (Yeandle *et al.* 2006). The Chinese population is the most disparately spread group, as well as being the only ethnic group that lives in both urban and rural circumstances (Garner and Bhattacharyya 2011).

Among ethnic minority households, 19 per cent report living in poor-quality environments, compared to 14 per cent of white households (DCLG 2013). The majority of ethnic minority communities live in cities or large conurbations, often in particularly disadvantaged areas, so are less likely to experience the advantages of green space, which has been identified in Chapter 2 as having a positive impact on health.

Social justice and equity
Deprivation and poverty

Poverty means having an income of less than 60 per cent of the median household income (Institute of Race Relations n.d.). It is more widespread in all BME groups than among most white populations, with people from ethnic groups getting paid a lower wage than their white counterparts (Barnard and Turner 2011). There are commonalities within the experience of some people from ethnic backgrounds, but differences within and across ethnic groups need to be recognized.

Levels of poverty vary across ethnic groups, with nearly three-quarters of seven-year-old Bangladeshi and Pakistani children living in poverty compared to just over half of those from Black backgrounds and one-quarter of white households in 2010 (Institute of Race Relations n.d.). London's Poverty Profile (2013) found that:

- the proportion of Black Africans living in poverty is twice as high as the white population, and still higher among Bangladeshis and Pakistanis, but that the proportion of Indians is no different from the proportions of white groups
- more than half of all people living in poverty in London are from BME backgrounds
- work rates in London are lower for BME groups, with 20 per cent of white adults of working age being out of work, compared with 60 per cent of Bangladeshis and 40 per cent of Pakistanis
- Bangladeshi and Pakistani workers are much more likely to be on a low wage than whites or Black Caribbeans.

This study highlights that lower work rates do not fully explain the high levels of poverty experienced by ethnic minorities, accounting for only one-third of poverty differentials. It is supported by a report by the Black Southwest Network (BSWN 2012), which identifies that the proportion of individuals who live in low-income households is:

- 20 per cent for white people
- 30 per cent for Indians and Black Caribbeans
- 50 per cent for Black Africans
- 60 per cent for Pakistanis
- 70 per cent for Bangladeshis.

Outside London, Gypsy, Traveller and Roma communities experience some of the poorest health, as identified, for example, in Leeds (Leeds City Council 2013).

The experience of poverty can differ across the country. Athwal *et al.* (2011) found that Bangladeshis, Afro-Caribbeans and whites all reported difficulties in living on low incomes, but Afro-Caribbeans' experience was much more isolating, because they did not have the same family networks that the other two groups had.

Poverty is experienced differently by gender, as well as ethnicity. A study in Newcastle (Warburton Brown 2011) found that:

- Pakistani and Bangladeshi women are particularly deprived, with large households, low educational achievement, low rates of employment and poor physical and mental health.

- Black African women also have low incomes and low employment rates, but that their educational levels and health are similar to the national average.
- Indian women have high unemployment rates, but that they come from a range of backgrounds, with some prosperous and others not.

Crime

Black and ethnic minorities have very different experiences of crime when compared with the white population, both as victims and as suspects or perpetrators. With regard to the former, racist and religiously aggravated incidents recorded by the police have decreased from 2005 to 2010 by 26 per cent. The risk of being a victim of personal crime was higher for BME groups than for whites, with those from mixed backgrounds experiencing the highest levels (MoJ 2011). People from Black and Asian groups are more likely to be homicide victims, with the majority of incidents being perpetrated by someone from the same ethnic group (88 per cent of white victims, 78 per cent of Black victims and 60 per cent of Asian victims) (*ibid.*).

A police officer has powers to stop someone at any time to ask what the person is doing, why they are in an area and where they are going (Gov.UK n.d.). These powers have been used disproportionately against certain groups, in particular ethnic minority people, with Black people being six times and Asians being twice as likely to be stopped and searched by the police in England and Wales (Equality and Human Rights Commission 2010). The explanation that is often put forward that Black people are more involved in crime is not justified by the evidence. Indeed, the evidence suggests that racial discrimination seems to be the reason for being stopped by the police (*ibid.*).

From 2005 to 2010, there was a decrease in the number of arrests of white people across England and Wales, but an increase in the arrest rates of Black and Asian people (increases of 5 per cent and 13 per cent respectively). Black people were arrested 3.3 times more than white people in 2009/2010. However, conviction rates were higher for white than Black or Asian groups (81 per cent for white, 74 per cent for Black and 77 per cent for Asian) (MoJ 2011).

EFFECTIVE INTERVENTIONS

Build healthy public policy

Mental health policy and general public health policies have already been discussed. Any policy relating to children and young people is also of relevance here, but among the most important policies for BME groups are those relating to equality and equity. Many of the essential ideas are echoed in guidance for health services that explicitly state that there must be equity and no discrimination, as mentioned in Chapter 5.

The UK Government's recent plan to tackle hate crime (HM Government 2012b) identifies the following three elements:

- Preventing hate crime – by challenging the attitudes that underpin it, and early intervention to prevent it escalating.

- Increasing reporting and access to support – by building victim confidence and supporting local partnerships.

- Improving the operational response to hate crimes – by better identifying and managing cases, and dealing effectively with offenders.

Austerity measures, with their impact on housing, benefits, education and so on, will impact on young BME people, along with anti-migration attitudes and culture. Policy that addresses these issues can therefore have great impact on BME health and well-being. This may include improving the material circumstances of BME mothers by increasing their overall household incomes and ensuring better access to the income, for example following Oxfam's recommendations by supporting BME savings groups or ensuring that child-related benefits are paid into accounts in the mothers' names (Warburton Brown 2011).

Strengthen community action

A recurring theme in the literature about BME populations is the ongoing need to engage with individuals and communities at a personal level, to ensure that people's needs are heard and addressed. Community-led approaches that recognize the way attitudes are culturally constructed can significantly reduce stigma and increase levels of optimism. These local approaches can prove more effective than some top-down, national initiatives (Knifton *et al.* 2010). This is the case from addressing crime (Cunningham and Drury 2002) to working with carers (IRISS 2010) to addressing the needs of people with mental health problems (Knifton *et al.* 2010).

In 2005, the Department of Health took a community-development approach to tackling race and mental health issues, in recognition of the disparities that BME people experience (DH 2005). As a result, funding was found to employ 500 community mental health development workers for three years, although local NHS bodies were left to find funding after this, which only happened on an ad hoc basis. However, some work was evaluated very positively, such as Making Voices in Bradford, a BME mental health project that provided individual support, peer group support and a signposting and information resource, as well as developing networks, partnerships and research (Thomas *et al.* 2006).

Examples of local community engagement include local credit unions, which provide the two-fold advantages of increasing financial opportunities as well as promoting community engagement. Creating credit unions and similar for BME communities has been suggested as a way of improving opportunities to save and access finances, along with providing advice on finance and maximizing the take-up of child-related benefits (Warburton Brown 2011). This approach can be important in supporting organization within communities and reducing financial exclusion (Howard 2005). It has been identified as particularly important for all low-income communities, including those with specific mental health issues, where community involvement can have wide-ranging benefits (Mandiberg 2012).

For particular groups of people there may be appropriate third-sector or community interventions. For example, there is now a 24-hour national helpline that children at risk of female genital mutilation can call (NSPCC 2013).

Develop personal skills

Research with BME women (Warburton Brown 2011) suggests a whole range of services that grassroots organizations are in a position to support, including addressing poor English and numeracy and improving self-confidence.

Lau, Black and Sturdy (2008) provide a number of local examples of ways that personal skills can be promoted:

- active outreach to improve engagement with services that provide skill development
- mental health forum developed and facilitated by a Turkish-speaking learner, with group members deciding topics and areas of interest to be discussed, including immigration, stigma and discrimination, citizenship, and strategies to manage mental health distress in learning environments
- vocational services providing short courses in creative subjects, including dance, drama and music
- employing local BME women as classroom assistants and tutors.

Create supportive environments

A key element of reducing the inequalities that BME groups experience, which impacts hugely on their mental health and well-being, is improving the material circumstances of these populations and the racism that underpins the experience of most ethnic minority people. Some of these measures are strongly linked to building healthy policy. Racism can be tackled in many different settings, including schools, health services and the workplace. This can be aided by reporting of race and hate crime, including the recording and subsequent action by local authorities, such as is done in Newcastle City Council, Allerdale Borough Council and Brighton and Hove City Council (with details available on the council websites).

Reorientate services

Many ideas and issues around reorientating health and social services have already been covered in previous chapters and apply equally here. However, there are some that are of more relevance to the BME community. For instance, the following examples of good practice have been identified in mental health services: taking a client-centred approach to understanding the most appropriate method of offering counselling; using therapies that are culturally relevant to people; offering advocacy to support dealing with statutory agencies; and providing guidance on dealing with racism (Fernando 2005).

Along with the general requirement to ensure that there is no discrimination against BME groups, several guidelines reinforce the idea of equitable access to services, which should be culturally appropriate; for example: 'Ensure that children, young people and adults from black and minority ethnic groups who self-harm have the same access to services as other people who self-harm based on clinical need and that services are culturally appropriate' (NCCMH 2012b, p.107). Potential language barriers are also included in guidelines, which suggest that information should be provided in the client's preferred language and that psychological interventions should be carried out in the preferred language or with an independent interpreter (e.g. *ibid.*).

Racism, discrimination and insensitivity to cultural differences can occur within the health service (NCCMH 2011b). There are particular groups (for example, Afro-Caribbean groups) who seek help much less often than others and also access services later, so are more likely to need crisis treatment. Another barrier to accessing community care highlighted by service users was the stigma and negative attitudes associated with their diagnosis and treatment.

It is possible that where there are access problems for adults, they also affect access for their children. There are also issues around the fact that children may be expected to interpret for their parents.

For one particular group of people – those who have undergone female genital mutilation – recommendations to services include supporting those affected, treating it as a child protection issue, systematically collecting and using information (including reporting cases), holding professionals to account (after assuring they have the appropriate powers to act), and increasing public awareness (RCM *et al.* 2013).

Measuring quality and equity

Measuring quality and equity needs to be done with particular attention to cultural differences. Health Equity Audit (HEA) has already been mentioned as a key tool in reviewing the inequities in the causes of poor health and accessibility to appropriate and effective service. It offers an ideal opportunity to identify and readdress race inequalities within services. For example, NICE (2006) describes a number of applications. In Luton, a smoking cessation audit found that ethnicity data were incomplete: data were not collected using the standardized national categories, so, for example, particular ethnic groups were not identified, and the category 'mixed' was not defined. As a result, no comparisons of the use of smoking cessation services by certain ethnic groups, and no conclusions about whether the service was delivering an equitable service, could be made. In Huddersfield, an HEA of mental health service use and provision did have appropriate data, although it identified a need for more accurate recording. A gap was found in services to detect post-natal depression among South Asian women. Attendance by ethnic minority groups was found to be low at outpatient clinics, and this led to the recommendation that services needed to be redesigned to be more appropriate, effective, accessible and culturally sensitive.

PRINCIPLES INTO PRACTICE

The subject of young BME groups was chosen as an example of a group within the population. This application of public health analysis has been difficult partly because of the diversity within this group. The holistic nature of health and well-being (our first principle) means that it is centrally linked with cultural and identity issues that are complex for BME groups. In addition, for a young BME person, the probability of living in poverty, with its associated risks to mental health and well-being, is high. According to our second principle, such 'determinants of health' must be addressed. This chapter has tried to signpost effective practice where it is known, but has also uncovered the dearth of information about both need and interventions in many aspects. Clearly, involving communities, users and carers (our fourth principle) is a vital part of the way forward in addressing this issue.

Chapter 9

EXTENDED CASE STUDY

IMPROVING MENTAL HEALTH AND WELL-BEING IN PEOPLE WITH LONG-TERM CONDITIONS

KEY POINTS

- A total of 58 per cent of over 60 year-olds have a long-term condition, compared to 14 per cent of people under the age of 40, although the percentage of young people with a diagnosis is rising.

- People with long-term conditions are at risk of social isolation and intolerance: community and group interventions are one way to address this.

- Maintaining people with long-term conditions in their own home, particularly as they get older, is now seen as increasingly important: housing, mobility and support for carers are all of critical importance in achieving this, together with medicine management, health literacy and integrated services.

- Personal behaviours that affect physical health are likely to impact on long-term conditions and associated poor mental health.

- Long-term conditions and consequent poor mental health are closely associated with deprivation: ameliorative measures include tackling fuel poverty.

INTRODUCTION

This is the last of our case study chapters. Here we look at mental health and well-being issues for people with long-term conditions. A long-term condition is a health problem that cannot be cured but can be controlled by some form of treatment, medication or otherwise. As with the other two case studies, the sequence of headings from Chapter 2 ('Wider determinants'), Chapter 3 ('Life circumstances') and Chapter 4 ('Personal behaviours') is used wherever relevant. The final part of the case study uses the headings shared by Chapters 5 and 6 to discuss effective interventions.

A chronic physical health problem can both cause and exacerbate depression: pain, functional impairment and disability associated with chronic physical health problems can greatly increase the risk of depression in people with physical illness. People with diabetes, hypertension or coronary artery disease are twice as likely to suffer from mental health problems as the general population; people with chronic obstructive pulmonary disease (COPD) or cerebrovascular disease are three times more likely to suffer from mental health problems. Once someone has two or more long-term conditions, the likelihood of experiencing depression is increased sevenfold (DH 2011d). Generalized anxiety disorder and obsessive compulsive disorder are also common among people with chronic physical health problems (NCCMH 2011b).

The causal relationship between mental and physical health is a two-way process (Naylor *et al.* 2012). Depression increases the risk of the onset of coronary heart disease (Benton, Staab and Evans 2007) and can also exacerbate the pain and distress associated with physical illnesses and adversely affect outcomes, including shortening life expectancy. People with severe mental illness are at greatly increased risk of coronary heart disease, diabetes and respiratory disease and have higher rates of obesity (Brown, Inskip and Barraclough 2000; Cohen and Phelan 2001; DH 2006b; Nocon 2004). There is evidence to show that those with mental illness are likely to have physical illnesses undiagnosed, unrecognized and poorly managed (Cohen and Phelan 2001).

When a person has both depression and a chronic physical health problem, functional impairment is likely to be greater than if a person has depression or the physical health problem alone. The presence of a physical illness can complicate the assessment of depression, and some symptoms, such as fatigue, are common to both mental and physical disorders (NICE 2009b).

The situation is complicated by the fact that a mental health condition can itself be a long-term disabling condition. For example, worldwide, it has been estimated that schizophrenia falls into the top ten medical disorders causing disability, not only because of the symptoms of the condition but because of the side effects of medication and social factors such as isolation, poverty and stigma (NCCMH 2010b).

WHO IS AFFECTED?

There are approximately 15 million people with long-term conditions, of whom more than a quarter have a mental health problem (NICE 2012b); people with mental health problems are up to twice as likely to report long-term illness or disability (Singleton *et al.* 2002). Some 30 per cent of deaf people using British Sign Language have mental health problems, mainly anxiety and depression (Mental Health Foundation 2007).

Long-term conditions can affect people of any age, sex or ethnic group and can increase the risk of mental health problems in any of them. However, there can be differences between groups in terms of the scale of the effects or the complications around diagnosis and recognition of the problems.

Across the lifespan
Family history

Genetics play a significant role in many long-term conditions, such as heart disease (e.g. Simon and Rosolova 2002) and diabetes (e.g. McCarthy and Zeggini 2009). The importance of taking a family history has been enshrined in the inevitability of being questioned about it at most medical encounters, and reflects the impact that genetics has on illness.

Young people

There is an increasing prevalence of long-term conditions in young people, with one recent study finding that 15 per cent of all 11–15 year-olds have been diagnosed with one, the commonest being asthma (HBSC 2011).

Children and young people with physical disabilities and serious or chronic illness are twice as likely to develop psychological problems as those without (CAMHS Review 2008). They are more likely to have emotional or behavioural problems than other children (NICE 2009e). Unfortunately, when a child exhibits challenging behaviour, it is sometimes hard to recognize additional mood problems or depressive conditions (NCCMH 2005). Depression or mood disorders may also be missed in adolescents with physical disability who have complex endocrine diseases, developmental disorders, autism or Asperger's syndrome (*ibid.*).

The CAMHS Review (2008) found several reasons why physically disabled and chronically ill children did not always receive the support and care they required, including:

a lack of CAMHS involvement on paediatric wards (paediatric liaison service); differences in the culture, structures and working practices of medical staff dealing with physical disorders and those dealing with mental disorders; a tendency to overlook the impact of physical illness on mental health and vice-versa; a lack of expertise; and difficulties in co-ordinating services where child mental health and paediatric services fall under different employing trusts, which is the case in many areas of the country. (*ibid.*, p.82)

About 30 per cent of cases of depression in young people recur within five years. Social factors, including physical illness and disability, are known to affect the likelihood of either a continuing depressed state or a relapse (NCCMH 2005).

Younger people with long-term conditions are less likely to play an active role in treating or managing their condition than older people (Ipsos MORI 2011).

Adults

Depression is approximately two to three times more common in patients with a chronic physical health problem than in people who have good physical health and occurs in about 20 per cent of people with a chronic physical health problem (NCCMH 2009).

Older people

The prevalence of long-term conditions is strongly related to age: 58 per cent of over 60 year-olds have a long-term condition, compared to 14 per cent of people under the age of 40 (NICE 2013b). Changing demographics leading to increased ageing will result in a greater proportion of the population having a long-term condition (DHSS&PS 2012b).

Older people who self-harm have high rates of physical ill health as well as social isolation and depression and, although older people are less likely to self-harm, the consequences are often more serious (including being fatal) (RCPsych 2010). In older men, physical illness and disability are factors often associated with high risk of repetition of self-harming behaviour (NCCMH 2004c).

Life circumstances

As in the suicide case study, the headings in this subsection broadly follow the order of those in Chapter 3.

Black and Minority Ethnic groups

The consequences of poor long-term health are worse for BME groups (Harriss and Salway 2008). Those from Pakistani, Indian and Bangladeshi origin are significantly more likely to be diagnosed with diabetes, and Pakistani and Indian groups are more likely to be admitted to hospital with coronary heart disease compared to the general population (Follett 2011). Because of the increased risk of many chronic diseases, particularly heart disease and diabetes, for BME populations, which are associated with obesity, NICE (2014) recommends that interventions should be triggered at lower body mass index levels for these groups.

The immediate family is the main source of care for those with long-term conditions and therefore has a major impact on the outcomes, but understanding how this affects BME people is difficult, because household composition varies considerably (Salway *et al.* 2007). As with abuse (Wellock 2010), people from ethnic minorities are under pressure to hide ill health and appear 'normal'. Both having a long-term condition and being part of a BME group are associated with much reduced chances of employment, which increases the chances and risks of living in poverty (Salway *et al.* 2007). As discussed in Chapter 2, these are risk factors for mental health problems.

Bullying

Disabled children experience a very high incidence of bullying, particularly those with learning disabilities, despite the legal duties on schools to eradicate the harassment and discrimination of disabled people (Mepham 2010). These children tend to be silent about their experiences, and so the high levels of support that they need are not recognized, which leaves them excluded and 'shut out' from society (Phelan, Stradins and Morrison 2001).

As for hostility, harassment and abuse, which affect people of all ages, there is little robust data about the numbers of incidents, nor how BME groups compare with others (Hoong Sin *et al.* 2009). The impact of this targeted violence is profound, with a wide range of adverse implications for physical, emotional and sexual health. Disabled people often respond by using an avoidance or acceptance coping mechanism, which is exacerbated by agencies advising them to avoid risk situations (*ibid.*).

Care homes

There are known issues surrounding the diagnosis of sensory impairment or other physical disability among those in care homes, where many residents are already older with serious health problems (NICE 2013b). Mild but progressive sight and hearing losses are a common feature of ageing and may go unnoticed for some time, but can have serious effects in terms of a person's communication, confidence and independence.

Carers

Chapter 3 identified a range of issues relevant to caring. The majority of caring is of people with an impairment, a mental health problem or long-term physical health condition. In England, approximately 1.8 million people are employed in the care and support workforce and about 5 million people care for a friend or relative without pay. It is estimated that 76 per cent of older people will need support and care at some point (HM Government 2012a).

The NHS Mandate (DH 2013d) identifies that people with long-term conditions and their carers need to have improved personalization and coordination of care, as well as support for both the sufferer and their carers.

Caring can have an unfavourable impact on the emotional, mental and physical health on those providing it, and with people with long-term conditions, it is inevitably a long-term commitment (DHSS&PS 2012b). About half of carers are of working age, which can have a major impact on their employment prospects (Yeandle *et al.* 2012).

The people who become carers are often family members, who may themselves be older, such as partners, with a condition themselves, or may be young offspring (DHSS&PS 2012b). Services for parents may not be accessible to those with physical disabilities (Katz *et al.* 2007).

There can be particular problems when a young person is caring for a parent with a chronic illness. For example, safeguarding concerns arise when such a person self-harms daily by cutting to manage difficult emotions about their circumstances (NCCMH 2012b).

Homelessness

Beadle-Brown *et al.* (2012) looked at research with seldom-heard groups who have long-term conditions and found none focused on homelessness. However, it is well reported that homeless people are not healthy, with one charity finding that 43 per cent of their homeless clients had a physical illness and 49 per cent had a mental health problem (St Mungo's 2008). Taylor *et al.* (2012) identify homelessness as being 'characterised by tri-morbidity: physical ill health, mental ill health and substance abuse' (p.2).

Looked-after children

There is limited information about the numbers or characteristics of disabled children who meet the British legal definition of 'looked-after' children. Often these children are placed in hospital or adult residential settings (McConkey *et al.* 2004). When placed in other, more age-appropriate, residential accommodation, it is often out of the local authority area (Beresford and Cavet 2009). However, many disabled children spend their childhood away from home, with many spending most of their time in unofficial 'care' (Morris 1997).

Offenders

Within the youth justice system, 25 per cent of young people have a learning disability and 30 per cent have a physical disability (Davis 2012). There is a higher incidence of long-term conditions in the offender population as a whole compared to the general population (RCN 2010). This relates partly to offenders having greater risk factors for physical illness, with 76 per cent of prisoners in Scotland being smokers, compared with 25 per cent of the general population, so being more at risk of CHD and COPD (Sharp, McConville and Tompkins 2011).

Refugees and asylum-seekers

Refugees and asylum-seekers experience harsh conditions before admission into the UK. They typically have poor health, much related to the preceding conditions of their life, including tuberculosis, hepatitis, nutritional deficiencies and, particularly, trauma. People may be left with long-term mental health problems, and hypertension and diabetes seem to be a legacy of those settling (Morris *et al.* 2009). It can then be problematic for refugees and asylum-seekers to access health care in Britain (Taylor 2009).

Social isolation and inclusion

People who have long-term conditions are more at risk of both social isolation and loneliness as a result of worklessness, limited mobility, lack of transport, poor relationships with carers, changing social roles, socially undesirable disabilities and states of emotional and psychological distress and dysfunction (Holley 2007). Physical dysfunction and social isolation are two key elements that affect social networks (family, friends and colleagues).

Despite the robust evidence base of research showing the impact of social isolation on morbidity and mortality, and the important impact it has on people with long-term conditions, little is currently done to promote social inclusion or prevent isolation and loneliness (Nicholson 2012). Although the process is not fully understood, social activity can be linked to reduced risk of physical disability in those living in the community (Robotham, Morgan and James 2011).

It is clear that people with long-term conditions are at risk of social isolation. They are at increased risk of further isolation given that they are a group who tend to be older and continue to age, another risk factor of social isolation. Some of this group then have the added hazard of living alone or with people other than a partner, such as children or extended family members, which increases loneliness (Russell 2009).

Veterans of the armed forces

Members of the armed forces have better than average health, and the majority continue to have relatively good mental health on leaving, with rates of depression or anxiety being similar to the rest of the population (Iverson *et al.* 2009). However, long-term mental health problems are experienced by a minority of veterans, with the consequences of heavy drinking – such as self-harm, suicidal thoughts and post-traumatic stress disorder – being identified as problematic (Woodhead *et al.* 2011). The latter has been associated with physical disorders, with arthritis associated in most studies, and conflicting data regarding diabetes, CHD and stroke (Qureshi *et al.* 2009).

Personal behaviours

Personal behaviours can exacerbate or improve both mental and physical health conditions and well-being. In this subsection we describe briefly some of the key behaviours with an impact on long-term conditions. Bearing in mind previous comments that long-term conditions in themselves can increase the likelihood of certain mental health conditions, such as depression, any behavioural changes that improve long-term conditions are likely to benefit mental health too.

Healthy eating

Poor eating habits are related to increased rates of obesity or being overweight. In turn, this has a significant bearing on the incidence of cardiovascular disease, diabetes and so forth (DH 2001). People who are overweight or obese are less likely to engage in physical activity, thus exacerbating the risk of ill health (HSCIC 2013b).

Physical activity

Lack of physical activity is related to a wide range of long-term conditions. Levels of physical activity decrease with age (HSCIC 2013b). In Chapter 4 we noted that physical activity has been found to benefit not only physical health but also mental well-being.

Alcohol

Alcohol has been shown to be potentially beneficial in moderate amounts, for example in cardiovascular disease. However, alcohol misuse has been associated with approximately 60 diseases. Given that long-term conditions are associated with older people, and the prevalence of alcohol intake declines with age, it may be less of an issue for this group. However, it has been identified that this decline is changing, and there are now increasing rates of alcohol consumption in older people (NCCMH 2011a).

Smoking

Stopping smoking has been identified as one of the most important preventive factors of many diseases such as cardiovascular disease and COPD (NICE 2013c). Tackling smoking is the best way to reduce inequalities in mortality.

WIDER DETERMINANTS

Shelter

Throughout the literature, housing is identified as being crucial for people's health generally and to their mental health in particular (Marmot 2010b). Many health conditions are affected by poor housing, and this becomes increasingly the case as people develop long-term conditions and get older and often frailer. There is a growing proportion of people with long-term conditions and older people who are owner occupiers, who may not have the resources to maintain their home or make the repairs and adaptations required to allow them to remain at home (Tinker *et al.* 2013). The draft Care and Support Bill (House of Lords and House of Commons Joint Committee 2012–2013) acknowledges the importance of housing to an individual's well-being and recognizes that local authorities have a critical role when it comes to ensuring people with extra needs are supported.

Maintaining people with long-term conditions in their own homes, particularly as they get older, is now seen as increasingly important, both in terms of their health, their own expectations and cost (All Party Parliamentary Group on Housing and Care for Older People 2011). For many people, remaining in their own homes and living independently is of huge importance, and resources are often needed to ensure this can happen. One element of this is ensuring that housing is adequate: 26 per cent of households with people over 60, many of whom will have long-term conditions, are defined as outside established standards of decency (Vass 2013).

Education

People living with a long-term condition are more likely to be disadvantaged with regard to educational opportunities (The Scottish Government 2009).

Among children and young people, some behavioural and emotional problems will be associated with physical or learning difficulty or disability. Children with these problems are likely to have difficulties with attending or engaging in school. This all comes under the broad phrase 'mental health needs', but the issue of whether these young people are also identified as having special educational needs can depend more on local provision and attitudes than on an accurate assessment of underlying needs (CAMHS Review 2008).

Income (employment and unemployment)

People living with a long-term condition are more likely to be disadvantaged with regard to employment (The Scottish Government 2009). Those with a limiting long-term condition are half as likely to be in paid employment as those without, and the situation is even worse for those with more than one condition (DH 2012c).

Not only do long-term conditions affect the likelihood of employment, but once in employment the impact of the conditions can lead to increased absence rates, as well as negatively affecting productivity (Naylor et al. 2012). This is particularly the case when depressive illness is one of the conditions affecting the individual (Druss, Rosenheck and Sledge 2000).

There are examples of occupational hazards in particular jobs actually causing long-term conditions, such as: mining or working in certain dusty conditions leading to respiratory disease; exposure to harsh cleaning agents leading to skin conditions; and heavy lifting jobs leading to musculoskeletal problems.

A stable ecosystem and sustainable resources
Environment

The environment in which people with long-term conditions live can have a major impact on their experiences. Although 79 per cent of people in England report that they are managing their condition, this varies from 66 per cent to 86 per cent across the country, with people feeling less supported in London, the Midlands and northern urban areas (DH 2012c).

Mobility is critical for many people with long-term conditions. One in five (approximately 4.5 million) households include somebody with a mobility problem, most of whom are aged over 60 years. Only 3.4 per cent of homes have the essential features to ensure accessibility for people with mobility issues, such as level access to the main entrance (Vass 2013).

Beard *et al.* (2009) suggest that living in an urban environment may have a significant impact on the ability of a person who has disabilities to remain independent and age actively, because of the negative street characteristics, such as crime. Disadvantaged neighbourhoods have a range of impacts on people with disability, including perceived safety (rather than actual crime rates) and the acceptability of being able to walk around the area. Clark *et al.* (2009) suggest that dangerous neighbourhoods 'get into the body' (p.162), which decreases an individual's mobility through a range of psychosocial and psychological processes.

The benefits to mental as well as physical well-being of green space were outlined earlier. Access to green space is often problematic for those with long-term conditions or disability. If they cannot easily get to green spaces, they will be unable to reap the full benefits of green space to both physical and mental well-being.

Social justice and equity
Deprivation and poverty

People with long-term conditions are more likely to come from poorer backgrounds, with clear links between long-term conditions, deprivation and other disadvantages, including unemployment (The Scottish Government 2009). Those from social class V have a 60 per cent higher rate of long-term conditions and a 30 per cent greater severity of conditions than those from social class I. Someone living in an affluent area is less than half as likely to have a long-term condition as someone living in a disadvantaged area (*ibid.*). The onset of multiple morbidities occurs 10–15 years earlier in those living in deprived areas than those in affluent areas (Barnett *et al.* 2012). The effect of co-morbidity on mental health is stronger when deprivation is also present, with more than half of people with more than two long-term conditions having signs of significant mental health problems. Naylor *et al.* (2012) suggest that this 'points to a three-way interaction between social conditions, mental health, and physical health' (p.6).

Many of the welfare reforms discussed in Chapter 6 have a major impact on anyone with a disability or long-term condition, with benefits for disabled people bearing 29 per cent of all cuts, although they represent only 8 per cent of the population. Those with the severest disabilities, who make up just 2 per cent of the whole population, will bear 15 per cent of the cuts (Duffy 2013). This has the potential of leaving some of the most vulnerable people in society, a group already predominantly living in poverty, in even more need (UNISON 2013).

Fuel poverty is a consequence of inadequate income and can lead to both morbidity and mortality, with excess winter deaths of 24,000 in 2011/2012 in England and Wales, many of which are attributable to the inability to pay fuel bills (DECC 2013). One study showed that more than 60 per cent of people with long-term conditions reported struggling to pay their bills, with almost 70 per cent wanting their homes to be warmer (Family Mosaic 2013). The effect of fuel poverty on health is well recorded; it has a significant impact on people's mental health (Liddell and Morris 2010). It has a particularly detrimental impact on people with long-term conditions (DECC 2013).

Crime

All disabled people, including people with long-term conditions, face intolerance and stigmatization, with one study showing that half of the disabled people surveyed had been targets of hate crime, of whom more than a third were the victims of a physical attack (Nocon 2004). Hate crime seems to relate to how 'different' an individual is perceived to be, with the impact for people with long-term conditions dependent on how visible their conditions are (Roulstone, Thomas and Balderston 2011).

Discrimination is much more common if people have a mental health issue (Berzins, Petch and Atkinson 2003).

Cunningham and Drury (2002) found that disabled people were almost twice as likely to be burgled as non-disabled people, and four times as likely to have property stolen from them with the use or threat of violence.

A national survey in the US (Rand and Harrel 2007) found that violent crime against people with disabilities was 1.5 times higher than the rate for people without disabilities. The incidence of rape was more than twice the rate, and women were found to be more at risk. More than half of all violent incidents against people with disabilities involved those with more than one long-term condition. Nearly one in five victims believed that they were a victim as a result of their disability, and it was perceived that about a third of the perpetrators were under the influence of either alcohol or drugs.

Domestic violence and disabled women is an area that has been overlooked by government policy in the UK (Radford, Harne and Trotter 2006). Disabled women experience a disproportionate level of abuse, including physical, sexual and material. Perpetrators are partners and ex-partners (37%), unknown (28%), parents (15%) and service providers (10%) (Schuller 2005).

Offenders are more likely to be from backgrounds of social disadvantage, as identified in Chapter 2, and so are disabled people. The criminal justice system is more likely to be able to detect vulnerable offenders, who are less adept at avoiding arrest or manipulating the system in their own favour (*ibid.*). This is more of an issue for young people with learning disabilities and mental health problems than for people with long-term conditions, who tend to be older and therefore less likely to offend, given that 15–24 year-old males are the most likely demographic group to commit crimes (Jansson 2007).

EFFECTIVE INTERVENTIONS

People's aspirations are increasing, with those with long-term conditions wanting to live at home independently for as long as possible, to exercise improved choice and control over access to appropriate person-centred care and support (All Party Parliamentary Group on Housing and Care for Older People 2011). Over the last decade, much work has been focused on developing suitable support. Again we discuss this in terms of the Ottawa Charter areas for action.

Build healthy public policy

Government policy on long-term conditions and government policy on mental health have in some ways developed along rather separate lines, although mental health is certainly an important part of long-term conditions policy and long-term conditions do get mentioned in mental health policy.

The relationship between austerity measures and mental health has been mentioned earlier. Changes in welfare payments have been shown also to give rise to particular problems for those with long-term conditions, who find themselves having to undergo increasing numbers of assessments. Cases have been documented of the stress caused by such a regime being associated with heart attacks or other physical deterioration (Stuckler and Basu 2013).

Strengthen community action

It is increasingly being recognized that people with long-term conditions and the local communities they live in need to be put at the heart of their services, a key element in ensuring the relationship between the public and professionals is one of equal and empowering partnership (Vass 2013).

Many projects work at a local level to provide opportunities for social interaction (Family Mosaic 2013). Interventions that have been found to be of particular help have been befriending, mentoring, Community Navigators and social group activities (Windle, Francis and Coomber 2011).

Community violence prevention interventions should address the perceived safety of people with long-term conditions, and not just focus on young people. Building social capital and social support should be central elements of such interventions (Clark *et al.* 2009). Some projects have been developed that focus on engaging people with disabilities in addressing crime from their own perspective, through disability forums, provision of safety advice and developing ways in which people other than the victim can report crimes (Schuller 2005).

People with physical disabilities can find social support and a sense of community through disability-specific online groups. Involvement in these online communities can have a positive impact on participants' well-being (Obst and Stafurik 2010).

Develop personal skills
Self-management

Self-management has long been seen as the most appropriate way of supporting people with long-term conditions wherever possible. Until recently, the focus has been on ensuring that individuals have the appropriate equipment and adaptations, such as stair-lifts, access ramps and emergency alarms (Vass 2013). More modern tools include the use of mobile phones, computers and television (Tinker *et al.* 2013). Increasingly, more sophisticated technology is being developed to enhance the experience of people with long-term conditions, in some cases transforming their lives.

A key element of supporting people with long-term conditions is aimed at educating them in self-management skills. It is important to emphasize that a significant element of self-management involves people learning about their conditions. Enhancing health literacy, as discussed in Chapter 6, can make a significant difference to people's lives. Increasingly, such education can be delivered over the Internet, via web-based learning, distance learning and user forums.

Maximizing self-management requires empowering patients so that they are not the passive recipients of care, but are confident enough to make decisions about their lives. One element of this is ensuring that people have both access to information on the management of their conditions, and the ability to understand and use that information appropriately. Differing literacy, comprehension and communication abilities need to be taken into account (DH 2012c). Several councils, government departments and third-sector organizations make available simple, clear language summaries of their publications.

People with long-term conditions often require emotional and psychological care to support the individual, their carers and the wider family, given the high levels of stress caused by the burden of morbidity. From a self-management perspective, this means support in accepting the illness, managing symptoms, maintaining personal motivation, adhering to treatment regimes, coping with difficult medical procedures, and adjusting to changing expectations and changes in behaviour and routines (Fellow-Smith *et al.* 2012).

The Expert Patients Programme has been developed for people with long-term conditions, to improve their quality of life, increase their confidence and help them manage their condition more effectively. It is based on the premise that individuals understand their conditions better than professionals. Courses are delivered covering topics such as dealing with pain, fatigue and depression, relaxation and exercise, healthy eating, communicating with family, friends and professionals, and planning for the future. A clear added advantage of the programme is the opportunity for reducing isolation: 'having access to self-managed programmes which encourage responsibility for health and well-being supports people to become re-engaged with the local community as productive citizens with meaningful activities, i.e., volunteering, education and employment' (Expert Patients Programme n.d., p.2).

Group-based peer support (self-help) programmes are recommended (NICE 2011b) for groups of patients with depression and a shared chronic physical health problem, to allow sharing of experiences and feelings associated with having a chronic physical health problem.

Personalization

Part of the wider agenda of self-management is personalization of services, where people entitled to health and social care are supported in making their own decision about how their allocated budget is spent (DH 2009b).

Managed personal budgets have been implemented more effectively with younger people with disabilities and long-term conditions. Older people have had more restricted opportunities, and their need for social contact and engagement in rewarding activity has been ignored. Vass (2013) found that people valued named and continuing personal support, flexibility, access to information, advice and advocacy, and assistance in planning care. Choice is seen as meaningless if there is little or no knowledge of the available options (DH 2006c).

People with long-term conditions are consistently clear about what they want, which includes being involved in their care, being listened to, and having access to relevant information, self-care support, appropriate services and care outside hospital where possible (DH 2012c).

Medicine management

There is limited research into interventions aimed at improving outcomes for people with long-term conditions, and what there is provides mixed evidence of the interventions' efficacy (Smith *et al.* 2012). Improved prescribing and adherence to medication regimes were found to be effective, particularly if targeted at risk factors or specific functional difficulties. Focusing on specific conditions was found to be more effective than addressing a wider set of conditions. Medicine management is an area that needs to be addressed, since between one-third and one-half of all medication prescribed for long-term conditions is not taken as recommended, and that 4–5 per cent of all hospital admissions are consequent of preventable, medicines-related conditions (Goodwin *et al.* 2011). Community pharmacists have a preventive role. For example, they can conduct a Medicines Use Review, a confidential appointment to check how a person is getting on with their medicine, make sure it is being taken as intended and find out any problems. This is useful particularly for people taking several prescription medicines or those who have a long-term illness.

Create supportive environments
Housing

Housing is a key element in providing appropriate support for people with long-term conditions, which has a major impact on well-being. There is an increasing emphasis on supporting people to live comfortably and independently in their own homes; Home Improvement Agencies have been identified to support people with long-term conditions to do so (DCLG 2011b). Schemes that may help include:

- housing services, including handyperson schemes, energy-efficient services and home improvement (Vass 2013)
- ensuring that advice is made available on housing options and on personal finances (House of Lords and House of Commons Joint Committee 2012–2013)
- safety, including falls prevention (Family Mosaic 2013; Fire Service n.d.), fire prevention actions (Fire Service n.d.) and ensuring vulnerable adults are not at risk of abuse (DH 2000). Many Fire and Safety Services offer home visits to advise on smoke detectors and other fire prevention actions.

Working in partnership across agencies is seen as fundamental to ensuring that vulnerable people have their housing needs met, which includes health, social care, benefits agencies and environment services, as well as housing (DHSS&PS 2012b). All of these groups have a part to play in developing appropriate legislation and policy, as well as practice (House of Lords and House of Commons Joint Committee 2012–2013).

Education and training

A range of educational provision is in place for children and young people who exhibit disruptive, antisocial and aggressive behaviour, hyperactivity, attention and concentration problems and emotional problems, some of which will be associated with a physical or learning difficulty or disability (CAMHS Review 2008).

Education is important for those involved in the care and service provision for people with long-term conditions. In terms of nursing, partnership and collaboration between the NHS and higher education institutions has been encouraged, to enable staff to build on competencies, often using non-traditional methods of learning (DH 2006a), as well as professional and academic courses (Hammond and Feinstein 2006).

From a co-production perspective, as identified in Chapter 6, training is ideally delivered to both staff and people with long-term conditions. The Health Foundation's Co-Creating Health programme found training teams rather than individuals most beneficial, particularly when supported by senior leaders (Newbronner *et al.* 2013).

Social justice and equity

Suggestions to improve deprivation for people with long-term conditions include:

- measures to deal with fuel poverty problems, which include addressing energy efficiency, income and energy prices (DECC 2013)
- money management, including advice on budgeting and eligibility for benefits (House of Lords and House of Commons Joint Committee 2012–2013).

Workplace

Advice is available (NHS Choices n.d.) on supporting people with long-term conditions. It includes practical steps, like making simple adjustments at work, listening to the employee, who may well know what they need, and ensuring clear communication. Occupational health departments and occupational therapists can provide information, assessments, specialist advice and information (BAOT n.d.).

Reorientate services

The stepped-care model, as described in Chapter 5, is particularly relevant to those with long-term conditions, ensuring that they receive appropriate levels of treatment (making full use of lower-level interventions before moving to higher levels). Other improvements can also be effected in primary and secondary care, as described in the following subsections.

Improvement of condition management in primary care

General practices monitor certain aspects of condition management as part of the Quality Outcomes Framework, introduced in Chapter 1. Managing conditions helps to stop more serious complications arising; for example, in patients with diabetes, poor management of insulin and glucose or inadequate checking of circulation can result in serious lower limb problems. Patients benefit physically from condition management, but additionally it can reduce unnecessary hospital admissions, which means that those with mental health conditions are not subjected to the stress associated with hospital admission. It is, however, recognized that mental health conditions may affect the way that a patient's physical condition can be managed in primary care.

Improved diagnosis of mental health conditions in those with long-term conditions

It has been increasingly accepted that chronic physical illness affects a person's well-being, functional abilities and quality of life, and can lead to depression and/or anxiety disorders. This can be a consequence of the long-term condition and may increase the perceived severity of physical symptoms, which then has a further negative impact on the person's psychological health (DH 2011d). The Department of Health (DH

2012c) recommends that people with a physical long-term condition should be assessed for the presence of depression and anxiety as part of their personalized care planning process. GPs can assess patients with long-term conditions for depression, using simple screening questions.

The difficulties surrounding diagnosis in certain groups, for example people with special educational needs, adolescents and children, were outlined earlier in the section 'Who is affected?'.

Appropriate level and type of treatment

This subsection focuses on interventions relating specifically to those with both mental health problems and long-term physical conditions. People with long-term conditions often have mental health conditions (particularly depression), and there is good evidence that treatment of such problems can reduce the need for GP appointments, hospital stays and outpatient appointments. Yet these people are rarely referred for psychological therapy (DH 2011d). NICE (2011c) now has specific recommendations for appropriate levels of care for those with chronic physical health problems and different severities of depression.

Social prescribing, described in Chapter 6, also clearly has potential to improve the well-being of people with long-term conditions, as well as those with medically unexplained symptoms (DH 2011d).

For patients with both mental health conditions and long-term physical conditions, there appears often to be a lack of a holistic approach to care, with mental health conditions treated in one place and physical problems elsewhere. For example, primary care services provide a vital service for adults with schizophrenia, who consult primary care practitioners more frequently and are in contact with primary care services for a longer cumulative time than patients without mental health problems. A small percentage of service users have all their mental health care needs provided by primary care; this includes monitoring, treatment and support for their mental health problems in collaboration with secondary care services. Most receive much, if not all, of their physical care from primary care. However, although most GPs regard themselves as involved in the monitoring and treatment of physical illness and prescribing for physical health problems, only a minority of GPs regard themselves as involved in the monitoring and treatment of mental health difficulties for people diagnosed with schizophrenia and even fewer GPs are involved in secondary care Care Programme Approach (CPA) review meetings (NCCMH 2010b).

Telecare and telehealth

Telecare is the use of sensors, alarms and other equipment to help people with long-term conditions to live independently for longer. An example is the use of a monitor that alerts services if someone has not returned to their bed at night after a certain amount of time has elapsed.

Telehealth aims to support people with long-term conditions by supporting them to monitor their condition and manage it in partnership with the service provider. It consists of equipment according to need, for example apparatus to measure blood pressure or oxygen levels, which is monitored by clinicians, who can then advise action.

Telecare and telehealth are seen as ways of supporting people at home and saving on the increasing costs of hospital admission (K. Taylor 2012). There are several other benefits: care is delivered closer to home, with fewer access problems due to geography; there is greater choice for patients; and unnecessary hospital admissions are potentially avoided (Digital Policy Alliance 2013).

In England, there are approximately 1.5 million pieces of telecare installed and about 5000 telehealth users, and the Department of Health has invested in an evaluation programme (DH 2012c).

User and carer involvement

Guidelines now usually stress the need for user and carer involvement. For example, the NICE guidelines for depression with a chronic physical health problem (NCCMH 2009) state:

> Treatment and care should take into account patients' needs and preferences. People with depression and a chronic physical health problem should have the opportunity to make informed decisions, including advance decisions and advance statements, about their care and treatment, in partnership with their practitioners... If the patient agrees, families and carers should have the opportunity to be involved in decisions about treatment and care. (p.7)

Integrated care

Although there is currently a major focus on developing a model of shared decision making within provision, many services are required to offer the full range of support required to ensure that people with long-term conditions live the best life they can. The Department of Health (DH 2012c) identifies that creating integrated generic care teams at a locality level, with key workers, is central to holistic provision. These teams need to be linked to the GP practice and include community services, associated health professionals, social services and community and specialist nurses. If the emphasis is on empowering patients, then co-production of care plans, through active participation of all, can ensure the delivery of appropriate and acceptable services.

Looked-after children are particularly in need of an integrated approach to their care. Children may have complex needs as a result of physical disability or impairment, learning disability or a long-term health condition. Complex needs can encompass physical, emotional, behavioural and health needs and may require help from a number of different sources (NICE and SCIE 2010, modified April 2013).

'Everybody seems to be talking about collaboration, co-production, mutuality and partnership,' say Entwistle and Cribb (2013, p.ii). However, they go on to suggest that there is still a significant gap between the aspiration of collaboration and the experience of people with long-term conditions. Truly person-centred care requires very different ways of thinking, which is not just about speaking to the recipients of care, but fully engaging with them. It requires an approach that empowers people, promotes their autonomy and builds on their expertise of their own life and conditions. It also requires professionals to be educated to understand an asset-based approach, which focuses on the strengths of individuals (Foot with Hopkins 2010).

Measuring quality and equity

Quality improvement strategies are an important element of the asset-based approach to service provision. However, they need to remain within the remit of this collaborative approach, and not fall into traditional ways of evaluating services, wherein 'success' is measured by how well people are managed according to clinicians' expectations (Cribb 2011) or effectively deny the patient any say in service delivery (Shortus et al. 2013). Indeed, some self-management programme evaluations are still concerned with patient compliance and behaviour change, as measured from 'objective' measures, without recourse to people's experiences (Pearson *et al.* 2007).

In terms of self-management programmes, there is an increasing amount of evaluative evidence available, although this has not yet been subject to systematic review. However, one comprehensive example of evaluation is the Health Foundation's Co-Creating Health improvement programme, which identified a range of factors of relevance to other programmes developed to support people with long-term conditions. These include ensuring that approaches to self-management behaviour change are long term that techniques like goal setting are acceptable to those being supported in self-management approaches, and that delivery in partnership changes the perceptions of both clients and clinicians (Wallace *et al.* 2012).

Social return on investment (SROI) (as discussed in Chapter 1) has huge potential for the evaluation of services for people with long-term conditions. A recent example is the use of SROI in East Lothian to evaluate the Care at Home service for people with physical disabilities, which showed that using the principles and practices of SROI led to an understanding of the importance of continuity of care, as well as the quality of food they were offered and social contact (Inglis 2012).

The Expert Patients Programme has been shown to be cost effective, with a demonstration of social return on investment, where for every £1 invested, £3–£6.09 has been shown to be saved through improving quality of life and reducing hospital admission (Expert Patients Programme n.d.; Kennedy and Phillips 2011).

Equity audits have shown that access to services is unequal, with a lack of resources and opportunities for people with long-term conditions coming from more deprived backgrounds (Vass 2013).

PRINCIPLES INTO PRACTICE

We have chosen long-term conditions as the subject for an extended case study because it is a medically defined group, and therefore provides an example of public health analysis in the context that is most readily accessed by planners and providers in the health care system. It is also an issue of growing importance in view of the demographic trends. The four principles we set out at the start of the book have been applied to this group. Using the holistic model of mental health and well-being (our first principle) means that someone with a long-term condition can be flourishing mentally if they are in the right environment. However, people with long-term conditions and sometimes associated disabilities are particularly vulnerable to changes in social welfare policy, which can affect their ability to have adequate housing, mobility and income. (Our second principle is that these wider determinants of health must be addressed.) The application of public health needs assessment and evidence of effectiveness (the third principle) indicates the need for a multi-agency approach to long-term conditions. In line with our fourth principle, the involvement of users, carers and communities is vital if we are to break the link between long-term conditions and social isolation.

Conclusion

A WHOLE SYSTEM FOR PUBLIC MENTAL HEALTH

The book takes a whole-system approach, recognizing the dialectic between individual and state, and personal and collective responsibility. We have tried to avoid too much emphasis on current policy, but provide evidence for people to draw their own conclusions. In doing this we aim to make current evidence, and in some cases debates, available to a wide range of people from the front-line of service delivery, through to strategic planners. Wherever possible we have signposted the practical implications.

At the time of writing, political change is in the air. This is partly the normal rhythm of the electoral process. But there is also the fact that, as Hunter put it in the context of the European Union, the UK, while a highly centralized state, has 'entered uncharted waters in respect of political devolution to the countries making up the Celtic fringe' (Hunter 2003, p.157).

In addressing mental health and well-being across the four countries currently forming the United Kingdom, we have recognized how different the policy environments are in relation to both NHS structures and arrangements; and the high-level approach to fiscal and welfare policy. So, although the four strategies for mental health have similarities, as discussed in Chapter 1, the context for their implementation is different, depending on the level of devolved decision making.

In England the statutory role of Health and Wellbeing Boards to produce Health and Wellbeing Strategies should provide a structural way of leading and developing work that addresses holistically the issues of mental health and well-being. GPs, whose strategic role is currently very important in England, are only too aware of the high proportion of people in their waiting rooms that experience mild to moderate mental health issues such as anxiety and depression. It is to their practical advantage, as well as ethically sound, to shape services that promote positive mental health and prevent the escalation of mental health problems. Yet also in England there is no national or regional structure to mitigate the effect of the current austerity approach to fiscal problems, and welfare reform that will reduce the quality of life for many, such as the people with long-term conditions discussed in Chapter 9.

The austerity measures themselves are likely to have a differential impact on different regions, within England and across the UK. Beatty and Fothergill (2013) estimate that the present welfare reforms will take nearly £19bn out of the economy, which is equivalent to about £470 a year for every adult of working age in the country. However, they also calculate that the worst-hit local authority areas lose about four times as much, per adult of working age, as the authorities least affected by the reforms. As a general rule, the more deprived the authority, the greater the financial hit. Asenova, Bailey and McCann (2013), in five case studies of local authorities in Scotland, found that local authorities do not have the adequate tools to assess the social impact of the changes. They also face the challenge of 'meeting the "here and now" while focusing on longer-term strategies in order to avoid exacerbation of current inequalities which will ultimately result in increased social, financial and economic costs' (p.5).

In this difficult environment it is more important than ever to fully realize the role of the whole workforce in promoting mental health and well-being. Despite the diverse nature of the three extended case studies (a rare event, a medically defined condition and a population group), there are roles for many parts of the workforce who would not normally see themselves as part of public health activity. In the following table we have summarized some of those roles. Although the table focuses on the three case study topic areas, some of the emerging themes are very widely applicable, for example maximizing the potential of front-line staff so that they consider every contact a mental health and well-being contact and offer advice and appropriate signposting where necessary.

THE WIDER WORKFORCE AND WHAT EACH SECTOR CAN DO IN
RELATION TO THE THREE EXTENDED CASE STUDIES

Suicide	Young BME groups	Long-term conditions
Social services		
Social workers, youth workers and life coaches have a significant role. Train front-line staff to recognize depression. Address risk factors such as child abuse and domestic violence. Provide day care/respite services, for benefit of patients and carers.	Report race and hate crime, including the recording and subsequent action by local authorities.	Provide equipment to aid self-management and independent living, for example stair-lifts, access ramps, emergency alarms, mobile phones, computers and TV. Participatory interventions, particularly those including social activity and support. Train front-line staff to recognize long-term conditions.
Local authority welfare rights units		
Money management, including advice on budgeting, use of credit unions and eligibility for benefits.	Money management, including advice on budgeting, use of credit unions and eligibility for benefits.	Money management, including advice on budgeting, use of credit unions and eligibility for benefits.

Local authority planning departments		
Ensure that new traffic systems do not split communities or lead to isolation. Erect/maintain physical barriers to access to high-risk venues such as bridges or cliff-tops. Erect signs there with contact details for services such as the Samaritans.	Strategically plan for social cohesion (to address the fact that one in ten ethnic minority people report living in neighbourhoods that are polluted and grimy, as well as having high reports of crime, violence and vandalism).	Plan the built environment sympathetically for people with disabilities/mobility problems. Ensure nuisance neighbours do not exacerbate stress (untidy land, illegal businesses run from home). Create an environment (not just built) that supports health and well-being.
Education departments and schools		
Address bullying and low educational aspiration. Teachers can receive awareness-raising training. Educate about self-esteem. Ensure access to health care professionals at school for adolescents, including those who have experienced general bullying and sexual abuse, those with learning disabilities and those who identify as lesbian, gay, bisexual or transgendered.	Recognize that BME children and young people tend to achieve higher levels of educational attainment than their white counterparts from similar backgrounds. Address poor English and numeracy. Support young people from BME groups and address racism in all contexts.	Education is important for those involved in the care and service provision for people with long-term conditions. Collaboration between the NHS and higher education institutions to enable staff to build on competencies, often using non-traditional methods of learning, as well as professional and academic courses. Effective occupational health for teachers with long-term conditions.

cont.

Suicide	Young BME groups	Long-term conditions
Housing		
Address standards of housing, and ensure adequate housing exists. Ensure advice is available on housing options and on personal finances. Measures to deal with fuel poverty problems, which include addressing energy efficiency, income and energy prices. Address home security and community safety principles – safer by design.	Ethnic populations make up a higher proportion of those households living in social housing. Need to ensure involvement of BME communities in developing housing policy, particularly around achieving community cohesion. Address home security and community safety principles – safer by design.	Coordination of adaptations and home repairs (including provision of handyperson service) to ensure independent living continues – for example, stair-lifts, ground-floor extensions, security adaptations and home safety measures, including interventions to prevent falls. Provide support on discharge from hospital. Provide housing advice, including support in moving to more suitable accommodation. Address fuel poverty problems, including energy efficiency, income and energy prices. At the strategic level, coordinate and support housing providers, social and voluntary services to address deficit in attractive and appropriate apartments.

Cultural and leisure services		
Provide meaningful physical and social activities.	Provide appropriate physical and social activities.	Provide accessible physical and social activities.

Environmental health		
Act to reduce noise nuisance or other environmental factors contributing to stress.	Act to reduce noise nuisance or other environmental factors contributing to stress.	Act to promote availability of healthy food in shops, restaurants and take-aways. Adapt homes for access needs through Disabled Facilities Grants. Act to reduce noise nuisance or other factors contributing to stress.

Trading standards and licensing		
Enforcement of legislation to prevent the sale of tobacco or alcohol to young people.	Enforcement of legislation to prevent the sale of tobacco or alcohol to young people.	Regulate loan sharks, unscrupulous credit providers and scams that target the vulnerable.

Drug regulation and management at all levels (including GPs, pharmacists, pharmaceutical companies and government)		
Reduce pack sizes of over-the-counter drugs (e.g. aspirin and paracetamol) to reduce severity of outcomes of deliberate overdose. Supervised methadone administration to improve compliance and reduce leakage to illegal drug market.	N/A	Medicine management to ensure that medication prescribed for long-term conditions is taken as recommended.

cont.

Suicide	Young BME groups	Long-term conditions
Home Office		
Address the needs of refugees and asylum-seekers, particularly around processes and length of time in detention. Improve the operational response to hate crimes – by better identifying and managing cases, and dealing effectively with offenders.	Challenge attitudes that underpin hate crime, and intervene early to prevent it escalating. Increase reporting of hate crime and access to support – by building victim confidence and supporting local partnerships. Improve the operational response to hate crimes – by better identifying and managing cases, and dealing effectively with offenders.	Address the needs of refugees and asylum-seekers, particularly around processes and length of time in detention. Improve the operational response to hate crimes – by better identifying and managing cases, and dealing effectively with offenders.
Ministry of Defence		
Address emotional and practical support needs of current and ex-service personnel.	N/A	Address emotional and practical support needs of disabled ex-service personnel.
Voluntary sector		
Crisis support (e.g. telephone helplines). Address emotional and practical support needs of ex-service personnel.	Address poor English and numeracy. Courses to improve self-confidence.	Provide advice on benefits system. Address emotional and practical support needs of people with long-term conditions.

Counselling for the bereaved. Activities that reduce social isolation, particularly in the older population.	Create credit unions and similar for BME communities to improve opportunities to save and to access finances.	Measures to deal with fuel poverty problems, which include addressing energy efficiency, income and energy prices. Money management, including advice on budgeting and eligibility for benefits.
Criminal justice (national and local levels)		
Awareness-raising (of mental health issues and suicide risks) for police and prison officers. Assessment of suicide risk in those in police custody; assessment/monitoring of risk in prison and in newly released prisoners.	Address institutional racism; for example, ensure that stop-and-search powers are not used disproportionately against BME groups.	Be aware that all disabled people, including people with long-term conditions, face intolerance and stigmatization, including increased risk of hate crime and physical attack. Effective occupational health for police staff with long-term conditions.
Coroner		
Collect right information and ensure it is used for learning lessons. Deal sympathetically with families.	Be aware of institutional racism.	Collect information if mental health issues are related to death.

In concluding, it may be useful to come back to an individual's experience. We have shown that there are many different factors in life that significantly affect an individual's mental health and well-being. These factors are not independent of one another, nor are they independent of the environmental and economic factors described in the previous chapter. We can illustrate this with the example of an older woman who smokes and lives alone in a deprived area with little scope for recreational or safe walking. Social isolation is not unlikely: she is no longer going out to work; she does not feel safe going out for recreation; she is more likely to be unfit because of smoking and to become physically even less fit because she is not taking exercise – all of these factors contribute to her feeling less happy or confident in herself and can lead to depression, making her even more unlikely to go out. While this is just an example, it is not an unusual example, and the growing number of older people in the population makes it likely that the scale of the problem will increase unless action is taken now.

The example above also helps to illustrate another important aspect of life and mental health: the vicious spiral in which circumstances adversely affect mental well-being and mental ill health adversely affects circumstances. So, for example, it is harder to get a job with a mental health problem, but joblessness exacerbates mental ill health. Another example is the way that physical health problems can contribute to mental health problems, but mental health problems can also make it harder to deal with the physical health problems.

On the other hand, a positive spiral effect can emerge if action is taken. For instance, if the woman in the example above is befriended and gains confidence to go out once a week, she may then start to gain social contacts and improve her physical fitness. In turn, this will make it easier for her to increase the amount of social contact she has.

For many of the issues presented in this book, there is already evidence of successful ways of addressing them. In most cases, evidence suggests that a multi-agency approach is essential. The interrelationship between the issues reinforces this idea. For instance, tackling the mental ill health caused by physical ill health means not only giving lifestyle advice and checking for depression in primary care (and treating if depression is identified), but also ensuring the local environment is suitable for outdoor exercise and providing appropriate council facilities. Similarly, addressing the mental health problems of looked-after children involves cooperative working between at least the education sector, social services and the health sector, to identify and treat problems and ensure access to appropriate services. The extended case studies about suicide, young BME groups and long-term conditions also stress the need for joint working across many sectors to deal with the multifactorial nature of the problems.

The four principles we set out in the Introduction, and reflected on throughout the book, suggest that we develop and appreciate positive steps at all levels:

- The individual, recognizing the holistic nature of mental health and well-being, which is central to a person's ability to make life choices.

- The region and country, because tackling many of the social, economic, political, cultural and environmental determinants of health and well-being requires action at this level.

- The organization, where the two key public health tools of assessing health care need in the population and applying systematically assessed evidence about what works can be best applied.

- The community, which is essential if we are to frame appropriate priorities, particularly in contested areas.

Times of change are also times of opportunity. The structural causes of inequalities in mental health and well-being have remained with us despite political change in the past. We hope that this book has provided both conceptual frameworks and practical evidence-based interventions, to make the most of opportunities to enhance mental health and well-being, particularly among the worst off, over the years to come.

REFERENCES

Abbott, P. and Williamson, E. (1999) 'Women, health and domestic violence.' *Journal of Gender Studies 8*, 1, 83–102.

Abdulcadir, J., Margairaz, C., Boulvain, M. and Irion, O. (2011) 'Care of women with female genital mutilation/cutting.' *Swiss Medical Weekly 6*, 140:w13137.

Abramowitz, J. S., Shwarz, S. A., Moore, K. M. and Klerman, G. L. (2003) 'Obsessive-compulsive symptoms in pregnancy and the puerperium: A review of the literature.' *Journal of Anxiety Disorders 17*, 4, 461–478.

Aceijas, C. (2011) *Assessing Evidence to Improve Population Health and Wellbeing.* Exeter: Learning Matters.

Acheson, D. (1988) *Public Health in England: The Report of the Committee of Inquiry into the Future Development of the Public Health Function Cmnd 289.* London: Her Majesty's Stationery Office (HMSO).

Action for Happiness (2013) *Good News, We're Slightly Happier. But Why?* London: Action for Happiness. Available at www.actionforhappiness.org/news/good-news-slightly-happier-but-why, accessed on 29 August 2013.

Adi, Y., McMillan, A. S., Killoran, A. and Stewart-Brown, S. (2007) *Systematic Review of the Effectiveness of Interventions to Promote Mental Wellbeing in Primary Schools. Report 3: Universal Approaches with Focus on Prevention of Violence and Bullying.* Warwick: The University of Warwick.

Age Concern (2007) *Improving Services and Support for Older People with Mental Health Problems: The Second Report from the UK Inquiry into Mental Health and Wellbeing in Later Life.* London: Age Concern.

Agree, E., Bissett, B. and Rendall, M. (2003) 'Simultaneous care for parents and care for children among midlife British women and men.' *Population Trends 112*, 29–35.

Aked, J., Marks, N., Cordon, C. and Thompson, S. (2009) *The Five Ways to Wellbeing.* London: Centre for Well-being, New Economics Foundation.

Alcohol Concern (n.d.) *Factsheet 17: Alcohol and Mental Health.* London: Alcohol Concern. Available at www.alcoholconcern.org.uk/assets/files/Publications/Mental%20health.pdf, accessed on 15 June 2012.

All Party Parliamentary Group for Drug Policy Reform (2013) *Towards a Safer Drugs Policy: Challenges and Opportunities Arising from Safer 'Highs'.* London: All Party Parliamentary Group for Drug Policy Reform. Available at www.drugpolicyreform.net/p/inquiry.html, accessed on 29 July 2013.

All Party Parliamentary Group on Housing and Care for Older People (2011) *Living Well at Home Inquiry.* London: Council and Care.

Allen, J. (2008) *Older People and Wellbeing.* London: Institute for Public Policy Research.

Allen, M. (2012) 'Domestic violence within the Irish Travelling community: The challenge for social work.' *British Journal of Social Work 42*, 5, 870–886.

Allen, R. (ed.) (1986) *The Penguin English Dictionary.* London: Penguin Books.

American Psychiatric Association (2013a) *Diagnostic and Statistical Manual of Mental Disorders, Fifth Edition.* Arlington, Virginia: American Psychiatric Association. Available at http://dsm.psychiatryonline.org, accessed on 20 April 2014.

American Psychiatric Association (2013b) *Major Depressive Disorder and the 'Bereavement Exclusion'.* Arlington, Virginia: American Psychiatric Publishing. Available at www.psychiatry.org/File%20Library/Practice/DSM/DSM-5/DSM-5-Bereavement-Exclusion.pdf, accessed on 30 July 2014.

Association of Public Health Observatories (APHO) (2007) *Indications of Public Health in the English Regions. 7: Mental Health.* York: APHO.

Appleby, L., Mortensen, P. B., Dunn, G. and Hiroeh, U. (2001) 'Death by homicide, suicide, and other unnatural causes in people with mental illness: A population-based study.' *The Lancet 358*, 2110–2112.

Appleton, S. and Molyneux, P. (2011) *Housing and Mental Health.* London: National Housing Federation/Mental Health Network/NHS Confederation.

Armstrong, R., Waters, E., Dobbins, M., Moore, L., *et al.* (2013) '*The impact of interactive knowledge translation strategies to support evidence-informed public health in local government.*' Paper presented at *FUSE (The Centre for Translational Research in Public Health) Conference*, Holland, 22–23 April, parallel session 7b. Tilburg: Tilburg University. www.tilburguniversity.edu/migration-temp/tranzo/hollandfuseconference/abstracts, accessed on 23 June 2014.

Asenova, D., Bailey, S. J. and McCann, C. (2013) *Managing the Social Risks of Public Spending Cuts in Scotland.* York: Joseph Rowntree Foundation. Available at http://www.jrf.org.uk/sites/files/jrf/public-spending-cuts-scotland-full.pdf, accessed on 23 June 2014. *[Copyright Glasgow Caledonian University.]*

Action on Smoking and Health (ASH) (2011a) *Fact Sheet: Smoking and Disease.* London: ASH.

ASH (2011b) *Fact Sheet: Smoking and Mental Health.* London: ASH.

Ash, M. and Mackereth, C. J. (2013) 'Assessing the mental health and wellbeing of the lesbian, gay, bisexual and transgender population.' *Community Practitioner 86*, 3, 24–27.

Aspinall, P. J. (2009) *Estimating the Size and Composition of the Lesbian, Gay, and Bisexual Population in Britain. Research Report 37.* Manchester: Equality and Human Rights Commission.

Aspinall, P. J. and Mitton, L. (2008) '"Kinds of people" and equality monitoring in the UK.' *Policy and Politics 36*, 1, 55–74.

Athwal, B., Quiggin, M., Phillips, D. and Harrison, M. (2011) *Exploring Experiences of Poverty in Bradford.* York: Joseph Rowntree Foundation.

Association for Young People's Health (AYPH) (2011) *Key Data on Adolescence.* London: AYPH.

Baldwin, M. L. and Marcus, S. C. (2006) 'Perceived and measured stigma among workers with serious mental illness.' *Psychiatric Services 57*, 3. Available at http://ps.psychiatryonline.org/article.aspx?articleid=91336, accessed on 22 March 2013.

Bambra, C. (2011) *Work, Worklessness and the Political Economy of Health.* Oxford: Oxford University Press.

Bansal, N., Bhopal, R., Netto, G., Lyons, D., Steiner, M. and Sahidaharan, S. P. (2014) 'Disparate patterns of hospitalisation reflect unmet needs and persistent ethnic inequalities in mental health care: The Scottish Health and Ethnicity Linkage Study.' *Ethnicity & Health 19*, 2, 217–239.

British Association of Occupational Therapists and College of Occupational Therapists (BAOT) (n.d.) *Long Term Conditions.* London: BAOT. Available at www.cot.co.uk/ot-helps-you/long-term-conditions, accessed on 24 February 2014.

Barlow, J., Tennant, R., Goens, C., Stewart-Brown, S. and Day, C. (2007) *A Systematic Review of Reviews of Interventions to Promote Mental Health and Prevent Mental Health Problems in Children and Young People.* Warwick: The University of Warwick.

Barnard, H. and Turner, C. (2011) *Poverty and Ethnicity: A Review of Evidence.* York: Joseph Rowntree Foundation.

Barnett, K., Mercer, S. W., Norbury, M., Watt, G., Wyke, S. and Guthrie, B. (2012) 'Epidemiology of multimorbidity and implications for health care research, and medical education: A cross-sectional study.' *The Lancet 380*, 9836, 37–43.

Barton, J. and Pretty, J. (2010) 'What is the best dose of nature and green exercise for improving mental health? A multi-study analysis.' *Environmental Science and Technology 44*, 10, 3947–3955.

Batty, E., Beatty, C., Foden, M., Lawless, P., Pearson, S. and Wilson, I. (2010) *The New Deal for Communities Experience: A Final Assessment.* Sheffield: Sheffield Hallam University/Department for Communities and Local Government.

Baum, F., MacDougall, C. and Smith, D. (2006) 'Participatory action research.' *Journal of Epidemiology and Community Health 60*, 10, 854–857.

BBC (2012) *Welfare Reform and Not Paying the Rent 24.11.12.* London: BBC (British Broadcasting Corporation). Available at www.bbc.co.uk/news/uk-20459252, accessed on 3 January 2013.

BBC (2013a) *Durham Research Finds Loan Companies 'Preying on Poor'.* London: BBC (British Broadcasting Corporation). Available at www.bbc.co.uk/news/uk-england-24583073, accessed on 18 January 2014.

BBC (2013b) *Panorama.* London: BBC (British Broadcasting Corporation), 15 July 2013.

Beadle-Brown, J., Ryan, S., Windle, K., Holder, J., *et al.* (2012) *Engagement of People with Long Term Conditions in Health and Social Care Research.* Canterbury, Kent: QORU (Quality and Outcomes of Person-centred Care Policy Research Unit).

Beard, J. R., Blaney, S., Cerda, M., Freyel, V., *et al.* (2009) 'Neighborhood characteristics and disability in older adults.' *The Journals of Gerontology: Series B 64*, 2, 252–257.

Beardslee, W. R., Bemporad, J. and Keller, M. B. (1983) 'Children of parents with major affective disorder: A review.' *The American Journal of Psychiatry 140*, 7, 825–832.

Beattie, A. (1991) 'Knowledge and Control in Health Promotion: A Test Case for Social Policy and Social Theory.' In J. Gabe, M. Calnan and M. Bury (eds) *The Sociology of the Health Service.* London: Routledge.

Beatty, C. and Fothergill, S. (2013) *Hitting the Poorest Places Hardest: The Local and Regional Impact of Welfare Reform.* Sheffield: Centre for Regional Economic and Social Research, Sheffield Hallam University.

Becares, L., Nazroo, J. and Stafford, M. (2011) 'The ethnic density effect on alcohol use among ethnic minority people in the UK.' *Journal of Epidemiology and Community Health 64,* 20–25.

Beecham, J., Bonin, E., Byford, S., McDaid, D., Mullally, G. and Parsonage, M. (2011) 'School-based Social and Emotional Learning Programmes to Prevent Conduct Problems in Childhood.' In M. Knapp, D. McDaid and M. Parsonage (eds) *Mental Health Promotion and Prevention: The Economic Case.* London: Department of Health (DH).

Beider, H. (2012) *Race, Housing and Community.* Chichester: Wiley-Blackwell.

Beider, H. and Netto, G. (2012) 'Minority Ethnic Communities and Housing: Access, Experiences and Participation.' In G. Craig, K. Atkin, R. Glynn and S. Chattoo (eds) *Understanding 'Race' and Ethnicity: Theory, History, Policy, Practice.* Bristol: The Policy Press.

Bennett, J. (2004) *Emotional Well-being and Social Support Study: An Overview.* Glasgow: University of Strathclyde.

Bentley, C. (2008) *Systematically Addressing Inequalities in Health.* London: Department of Health. Gateway Reference 10060.

Benton, T., Staab, J. and Evans, D. L. (2007) 'Medical co-morbidity in depressive disorders.' *Annals of Clinical Psychiatry 19,* 4, 289–303.

Beresford, B. and Cavet, J. (2009) *Transitions to Adult Services by Disabled Young People Leaving Out of Authority Residential Schools.* York: Social Policy Research Unit, University of York.

Berkman, L. F. and Kawachi, I. (2000) 'A Historical Framework for Social Epidemiology.' In L. Berkman and I. Kawachi (eds) *Social Epidemiology.* New York, NY: Oxford University Press.

Berliner, P., Nikkelsen, E. M., Bovbjerg, A. and Wiking, M. (2004) 'Psychotherapy treatment of torture survivors.' *International Journal of Psychosocial Rehabilitation 8,* 85–96.

Bernard, S. and Turk, J. (2009) *Developing Mental Health Services for Children and Adolescents with Learning Disabilities.* London: Royal College of Psychiatrists.

Berthoud, R. (1999) *Young Caribbean Men and the Labour Market: A Comparison with Other Ethnic Groups.* York: Joseph Rowntree Foundation.

Berzins, K. M., Petch, A. and Atkinson, J. M. (2003) 'Prevalence and experience of harassment of people with mental health problems living in the community.' *British Journal of Psychiatry 183,* 526–533.

Bick, D., MacArthur, C., Knowles, H. and Winters, H. (2002) *Postnatal Care: Evidence and Guidelines for Management.* Edinburgh: Churchill Livingstone.

Biddle, S. (2000) 'Emotion, Mood and Physical Activity.' In S. Biddle, D. Fox and S. Boutcher (eds) *Physical Activity and Psychological Wellbeing*. London: Routledge.

Biordi, D. L. and Nicholson, N. R. (2013) 'Social Isolation.' In I. M. Lubkin and P. D. Larsen (eds) *Chronic Illness: Impact and Intervention*. Burlington, VT: Jones and Bartlett Learning.

Bird, W. (2007) 'Natural greenspace.' *British Journal of General Practice 57*, 534, 69.

Black, C. (2008) *Working for a Healthier Tomorrow: Dame Carol Black's Review of the Health of Britain's Working Age Population*. London: TSO.

Black, C. and Frost, D. (2011) *Health at Work – An Independent Review of Sickness Absence*. Norwich: TSO.

Blouin, C., Heymann, J. and Drager, N. (2007) *Trade and Health: Seeking Common Ground*. Montreal: McGill-Queen's University Press.

British Medical Association (BMA) (2003) *Housing and Health, Building for the Future*. London: British Medical Association Board of Science.

BMA (2007) *Domestic Abuse*. London: British Medical Association Board of Science.

BME Leadership Forum (2013) *Engaging with BME Communities: Insights for Impact*. London: NHS Confederation.

Boardman, A. P., Hodgson, R. E., Lewis, M. and Allen, K. (1997) 'Social indicators and the prediction of psychiatric admission in different diagnostic groups.' *British Journal of Psychiatry 171*, 457–462.

Bolton, J. (2009) *The Use of Resources in Adult Social Care: A Guide for Local Authorities*. London: Department of Health.

Bonari, L., Pinto, N., Ahn, E., Einarson, A., Steiner, M. and Koren, G. (2004) 'Perinatal risks of untreated depression during pregnancy.' *Canadian Journal of Psychiatry 49*, 11, 726–735.

Booker, C. and Boice, M. (2007) *Employment and Inequality: Closing the Gap and Removing Barriers*. Brighton: Sussex Institute, University of Sussex.

Borrell, L. N., Diez Roux, A. V., Jacobs, D. R., Shea, S., *et al.* (2010) 'Perceived racial/ethnic discrimination, smoking and alcohol consumption in the Multi-Ethnic Study of Atherosclerosis (MESA).' *Preventive Medicine 51*, 3–4, 307–312.

British Psychological Society, The (BPS) (2012) *Truancy and Mental Health Problems*. Leicester: The British Psychological Society. Available at www.bps.org.uk/news/truancy-and-mental-health-problems, accessed on 29 May 2013.

Bradley, K. (2009) *The Bradley Report: Lord Bradley's Review of People with Mental Health Problems or Learning Disabilities in the Criminal Justice System*. London: DH Publications.

Bradshaw, J., Finch, N., Mayhew, E., Ritackallio, V. and Skinner, C. (2006) *Child Poverty in Larger Families*. York: Joseph Rowntree Foundation.

Brady, J. (2006) 'The association between alcohol misuse and suicidal behaviour.' *Alcohol and Alcoholism 41*, 5, 473–478.

Breakwell, C., Baker, A., Griffiths, C., Jackson, G., Fegan, G. and Marshall, D. (2007) 'Trends and geographical variations in alcohol-related deaths in the United Kingdom, 1991–2004.' *Health Statistics Quarterly, Spring*, 33, 6–24.

British Association for the Humanities and Social Sciences (2014) *If You Could do One Thing: Nine Local Actions to Reduce Inequalities.* London: The British Academy. Available at www.britac.ac.uk/policy/Health_Inequalities.cfm, accessed on 21 February 2014.

Brockington, I. F. (1996) *Motherhood and Mental Health.* Oxford: Oxford University Press.

Brooker, D. and Surr, C. (2005) *Dementia Care Mapping: Principles and Practice.* Bradford: University of Bradford.

Brown, G. W. and Moran, P. M. (1997) 'Single mothers, poverty and depression.' *Psychological Medicine 21*, 21–33.

Brown, J. (2009) *Skilled for Health: Evaluation of Pilot Programme, Gateshead.* Gateshead: Gateshead Primary Care Trust.

Brown, J. (2012) *Gateshead Housing and Falls Prevention: An Evaluation Report Prepared for Gateshead Housing and Falls Team.* Gateshead: Gateshead PCT and Gateshead Council.

Brown, J., Shassere, E. and Sengupta, S. (2005) *Health in Regional Public Policy: Using Assessment Techniques to Improve the Impact of Policy on Health.* Durham: HDA (Health Development Agency) and Durham University. Available at www.apho.org.uk/resource/view.aspx?RID=44254, accessed on 20 July 2014.

Brown, M., Friedli, L. and Watson, S. (2004) 'Prescriptions for pleasure.' *Mental Health Today*, June, 20–23.

Brown, S., Inskip, H. and Barraclough, B. (2000) 'Causes of the excess mortality of schizophrenia.' *British Journal of Psychiatry 177*, 212–217.

Brown, V., Clery, E. and Ferguson, C. (2011) *Estimating the Prevalence of Young People Absent from School due to Bullying.* London: National Centre for Social Research.

Brugha, T. S., Bebbington, T. E., MacCarthy, B., Sturt, E., Wykes, T. and Potter, J. (1990) 'Gender, social support and recovery from depressive disorders: A prospective clinical study.' *Psychological Medicine 20*, 1, 147–156.

Black Southwest Network (BSWN) (2012) *Poverty in Black and White.* Bristol: BSWN. Available at http://bswnsouthwest.wordpress.com/2012/08/03/a-new-approach-to-child-poverty, accessed on 21 November 2013.

Buck, D. and Frosini, F. (2012) *Clustering of Unhealthy Behaviours Over Time: Implications for Policy and Practice.* London: The King's Fund.

Buckner, L. and Yeandle, S. (2011) *Valuing Carers 2011: Calculating the Value of Carers' Support.* London: University of Leeds/Carers UK.

Burchardt, T. (2003) *Employment Retention and the Onset of Sickness or Disability: Evidence from the Labour Force Survey (LFS) Longitudinal Data Sets.* London: Department for Work and Pensions.

Burton, D. L., Duty, K. J. and Leibowitz, G. S. (2011) 'Differences between sexually victimized and nonsexually victimized male adolescent sexual abusers: Developmental antecedents and behavioral comparisons.' *Journal of Child Sexual Abuse 20*, 1, 77–93.

Butland, B., Jebb, S., Kopelman, P., McPherson, K., *et al.* (2007) *Foresight. Tackling Obesities: Future Choices – Project Report, Second Edition.* London: Government Office for Science.

Butler, V. (2007) *Young People's Experiences of, and Solutions to, Identity Related Bullying.* Cardiff: Barnardo's Cymru.

Butterworth, P., Leach, L. S., Pirkis, J. and Kelaher, M. (2012) 'Poor mental health influences risk and duration of unemployment: A prospective study.' *Social Psychiatry and Psychiatric Epidemiology 47*, 6, 1013–1021.

Cabinet Office (2010) *State of the Nation Report: Poverty, Worklessness and Welfare Dependency in the UK.* London: Cabinet Office.

Child and Adolescent Mental Health Services (CAMHS) Review (2008) *Children and Young People in Mind: The Final Report of the National CAMHS [Child and Adolescent Mental Health Services] Review.* London: CAMHS Review.

Campbell, C., Wood, R. and Kelly, M. (1999) *Social Capital and Health.* London: Health Education Authority.

Campion, J., Checinski, K. and Nurse, J. (2008) 'Review of smoking cessation treatments for people with mental illness.' *Advances in Psychiatric Treatment 4*, 208–216.

Caplan, G. (1961) *An Approach to Community Mental Health.* London: Tavistock Publications.

Care Quality Commission (2013) *Community Mental Health Survey 2013.* London and Newcastle: Care Quality Commission.

Carers UK (2004) *In Poor Health: The Impact of Caring on Health.* London: Carers UK.

Carers UK (2011) *The Cost of Caring: How Money Worries are Pushing Carers to Breaking Point.* London: Carers UK.

Carers UK (2012) *Facts about Carers 2012. Policy Briefing.* London: Carers UK.

Cattan, M. and Tilford, S. (2006) *Mental Health Promotion: A Lifespan Approach.* Maidenhead /New York, NY: Open University Press/McGraw-Hill.

Cattan, M., White, M., Bond, J. and Learmonth, A. (2005) 'Preventing social isolation and loneliness among older people: A systematic review of health promotion interventions.' *Ageing and Society 25*, 1, 41–67.

Centre for Mental Health (updated 2011) *Briefing 39: Mental Health Care and the Criminal Justice System.* London: Centre for Mental Health. Available at www.centreformentalhealth.org.uk/pdfs/briefing_39_revised.pdf, accessed on 12 May 2012.

Chambers Giant Paperback English Dictionary (1996) Edinburgh: Chambers, an imprint of Larousse.

Chartier, M. J., Walker, J. R. and Naimark, B. (2009) 'Health risk behaviors and mental health problems as mediators of the relationship between childhood abuse and adult health.' *American Journal of Public Health 99*, 5, 848–854.

Children's Society, The (2012) *Promoting Positive Well-being for Children. A Report for Decision-makers in Parliament, Central Government and Local Areas.* Leeds: The Children's Society.

Church, E. and Ryan, T. (n.d.) *Suicide Audit in Primary Care Trust Locations: A Whole Systems Approach – Supporting Evidence for a Primary Care Suicide Audit.* London: CSIP (Care Services Improvement Partnership), NIMHE (National Institute for Mental Health England), Department of Health.

Citizens Advice (2012) *Debt, Health and Wellbeing Survey.* London: Citizens Advice.

Clark, C., Rodgers, B., Caldwell, T., Power, C. and Stansfeld, S. (2007) 'Childhood and adulthood psychological ill health as predictors of midlife affective and anxiety disorders: The 1958 British Birth Cohort.' *Archive of General Psychiatry 64*, 6, 668–678.

Clark, C. R., Kawachi, I., Ryan, L., Ertel, K., Fay, M. E. and Berkman, L. F. (2009) 'Perceived neighborhood safety and incident mobility disability among elders: The hazards of poverty.' *BMC Public Health 9*, 162.

Clarke, N., Barnett, C., Cloke, P. and Malpass, A. (2007) 'Globalising the consumer.' *Political Geography 26*, 231–249.

Cohen, A. and Phelan, M. (2001) 'The physical health of patients with mental illness: A neglected area.' *Mental Health Promotion Update 2*, 15–16.

Colman, I., Murray, J., Abbott, R., Maughan, B., *et al.* (2009) 'Outcomes of conduct problems in adolescence: 40 year follow-up of national cohort.' *British Medical Journal 338*, a2981.

Commission for Healthcare Audit and Inspection (2007) *Count Me In: National Census of Inpatients in Mental Health Hospitals and Facilities in England and Wales.* London: Commission for Healthcare Audit and Inspection.

Committee on America's Climate Choices (2011) *America's Climate Choices.* Washington, DC: The National Academies Press. Available at www.nap.edu/openbook.php?record_id=12781&page=R1, accessed on 28 April 2013.

Community Development Cymru (2007) *National Strategic Framework for Community Development in Wales.* Powys: Community Development Cymru.

Condon, J. (2010) 'Women's mental health: A "wish-list" for the DSM V.' *Archives of Women's Mental Health 13*, 1, 5–10.

Contact a Family (2011) *Forgotten Families: The Impact of Isolation on Families with Disabled Children Across the UK.* Available at www.cafamily.org.uk/media/381636/forgotten_isolation_report.pdf, accessed on 12 January 2013.

Conwell, Y., Duberstein, P. R., Hirsch, J. K., Conner, K. R., Eberly, S. and Caine, E. D. (2010) 'Health status and suicide in the second half of life.' *International Journal of Geriatric Psychiatry 25*, 4, 371–379.

Cook, A. and Miller, E. (2012) *Personal Outcomes Approach.* Edinburgh: Joint Improvement Team.

Cooke, A., Friedli, L., Coggins, T., Edmonds, N., *et al.* (2011) *Mental Wellbeing Impact Assessment: A Toolkit for Wellbeing, Third Edition.* London: National Mental Wellbeing Impact Assessment Collaborative.

Cooke, A. and Stansfield, J. (2009) *Improving Mental Wellbeing through Impact Assessment: A Summary of the Development and Application of a Mental Well-being Impact Assessment Tool.* London: National Mental Health Development Unit.

Cooper, H., Arber, S., Fee, L. and Ginn, J. (1999) *The Influence of Social Support and Social Capital on Health: A Review and Analysis of British Data.* London: Health Education Authority.

Cooperrider, D. L. and Whitney, D. (2005) 'Appreciative Inquiry: A Positive Revolution in Change.' In P. Holman and T. Devane (eds) *The Change Handbook.* San Francisco, CA: Berrett-Koehler Publishers.

Cornaglia, F., Crivellaro, E. and McNally, S. (2012) *Mental Health and Education Decisions.* London: Centre for the Economics of Education, London School of Economics.

Cornah, D. (2004) *Feeding Minds: The Impact of Food on Mental Health.* London: Mental Health Foundation.

Cox, J. L. (1989) 'Postnatal depression: A serious and neglected postpartum complication.' *Bailliere's Clinical Obstetrics and Gynaecology 3*, 839–855.

Craig, P., Cooper, C., Gunnell, D., Haw, S., *et al.* (2011) *Using Natural Experiments to Evaluate Population Health Interventions.* London and Swindon: MRC (Medical Research Council).

Craig, P., Dieppe, P., Macintyre, S., Michie, S., Nazareth, I. and Petticrew, M. (2008) *Complex Interventions Guidance.* London and Swindon: MRC (Medical Research Council).

Cramer, R. J., McNiel, D. E. and Holley, S. R. (2012) 'Mental health in violent crime victims: Does sexual orientation matter?' *Law and Human Behaviour 36*, 2, 87–95.

Cribb, A. (2011) *Involvement, Shared Decision-making and Medicines.* London: Centre for Public Policy Research, King's College.

Crisis (2011) *Homelessness: A Silent Killer. A Research Briefing on Mortality amongst Homeless People.* London: Crisis.

Croudace, T. J., Kayne, R., Jones, P. B. and Harrison, G. L. (2000) 'Non-linear relationship between an index of social deprivation psychiatric admission prevalence and the incidence of psychosis.' *Psychological Medicine 30*, 177–185.

Cruse (Cruse Bereavement Care) (n.d.) *Children and Young People's Emotional Responses.* Richmond, Surrey: Cruse. Available at www.cruse.org.uk/Children/emotional-response, accessed on 30 July 2013.

Cunningham, S. and Drury, S. (2002) *Access all Areas: A Guide for Community Safety Partnerships on Working More Effectively with Disabled People.* London: Nacro.

Curtis, S. (2010) *Space, Place and Mental Health.* Surrey: Ashgate Publishing Limited. Available at www.ashgate.com/isbn/9780754673316, accessed on 20 July 2014.

Daniels, S. (2012) *Depression in Young People with Learning Disabilities: Identification and Accessing Support.* London: The Judith Trust.

Davies, H. T. O., Nutley, S. M. and Smith, P. C. (2000) *What Works? Evidence-based Policy and Practice in Public Services.* Bristol: The Policy Press.

Davis, L. (2012) *Children and Equality – Equality Evidence Relating to Children and Young People in England.* London: Office of the Children's Commissioner.

Department for Communities and Local Government (DCLG) (2010) *Effectiveness of Schemes to Enable Households at Risk of Domestic Violence to Remain in their Own Homes.* London: DCLG.

DCLG (2011a) *Community Spirit in England: A Report on the 2009–10 Citizenship Survey*. London: DCLG.

DCLG (2011b) *Laying the Foundations: A Housing Strategy for England*. London: DCLG.

DCLG (2012a) *Making Every Contact Count: A Joint Approach to Preventing Homelessness*. London: DCLG.

DCLG (2012b) *Working with Troubled Families: A Guide to the Evidence and Good Practice*. London: DCLG.

DCLG (2013) *English Housing Survey: HOUSEHOLDS. Annual Report on England's Households, 2011-12*. London: DCLG.

De Anstiss, H., Ziaian, T., Procter, N., Warland, J. and Baghurst, P. (2009) 'Help-seeking for mental health problems in young refugees: A review of the literature with implications for policy, practice and research.' *Transcultural Psychiatry 46*, 4, 584–607.

De Grace, A. and Clarke, A. (2012) 'Promising practices in the prevention of intimate partner violence among adolescents.' *Violence and Victims 27*, 6, 849–859.

Department of Energy and Climate Change (DECC) (2013) *Fuel Poverty: A Framework for Future Action*. London: TSO.

Devins, D., Bickerstaffe, T., Mitchell, B. and Halliday, S. (2014) *Improving Progression in Low-paid, Low-skilled Retail, Catering and Care Jobs*. York: Joseph Rowntree Foundation.

Department for Education (DfE) (2011) *Raising the Aspirations and Educational Outcomes of Looked After Children: A Data Tool for Local Authorities*. London: DfE. Available at www.education.gov.uk/childrenandyoungpeople/families/childrenincare/a00192332/raising-the-aspirations-and-educational-outcomes-of-looked-after-children-a-data-tool-for-local-authorities, accessed on 30 July 2013.

DfE (2013) *Statistical First Release: Pupil Absence in Schools in England, Autumn Term 2012 (SFR 17/2013)*. London: DfE.

DfE (n.d.) *Healthy Schools*. London: DfE. Available at www.education.gov.uk/schools/pupilsupport/pastoralcare/a0075278/healthy-schools, accessed on 16 December 2013.

Department of Health (DH) (1998) *Independent Inquiry into Inequalities in Health Report (Acheson Report)*. London: TSO.

DH (2000) *No Secrets: Guidance on Developing and Implementing Multi-agency Policies and Procedures to Protect Vulnerable Adults from Abuse*. London: TSO.

DH (2001) *National Service Framework for Diabetes: Standards*. London: DH.

DH (2002) *Dual Diagnosis Good Practice Guide*. London: DH.

DH (2003) *Health Equity Audit: A Guide for the NHS*. London: DH.

DH (2005) *Delivering Race Equality in Mental Health Care: An Action Plan for Reform Inside and Outside Services and the Government's Response to the Independent Inquiry into the Death of David Bennett. The Independent Inquiry into the Death of David Bennett*. London: DH.

DH (2006a) *Caring for People with Long Term Conditions: An Education Framework for Community Matrons and Case Managers.* Leeds: DH.

DH (2006b) *Choosing Health: Supporting the Physical Health Needs of People with Severe Mental Illness.* London: DH.

DH (2006c) *Our Health, Our Care, Our Say: A New Direction for Community Services. Cm 6737.* Norwich: TSO.

DH (2007a) *Lesbian, Gay and Bisexual (LGB) People from Black and Minority Ethnic Communities.* London: DH.

DH (2007b) *Mental Health Issues within Lesbian, Gay and Bisexual (LGB) Communities.* London: DH.

DH (2008) *End of Life Care Strategy: Promoting High Quality Care for Adults at the End of their Life.* London: DH.

DH (2009a) *Improving Health, Supporting Justice: The National Delivery Plan of the Health and Criminal Justice Programme Board.* London: DH.

DH (2009b) *Tackling Health Inequalities 10 Years On.* London: DH.

DH (2010a) *Practical Approaches to Co-production: Building Effective Partnerships with People Using Services, Carers, Families and Citizens.* London: DH. Available at www.thinklocalactpersonal.org.uk/_library/PPF/NCAS/Practical_approaches_to_co-production_12_November_2010_v3_ACC.pdf, accessed on 8 June 2013.

DH (2010b) *Recognised, Valued and Supported: Next Steps for the Carers Strategy.* London: DH.

DH (2011a) *Consultation on Preventing Suicide in England.* London: DH.

DH (2011b) *Improved Mental Health Therapies for Children.* London: DH.

DH (2011c) *Public Health in Local Government Factsheets.* London: DH.

DH (2011d) *Talking Therapies: A Four-year Plan of Action.* London: COI for the DH.

DH (2012a) *The Adult Social Care Outcomes Framework 2013/14.* London: DH.

DH (2012b) *Improving Outcomes and Supporting Transparency. Part 1: A Public Health Outcomes Framework for England 2013–2016.* London: DH.

DH (2012c) *Long Term Conditions Compendium of Information.* London: DH.

DH (2013a) *A Framework for Sexual Health Improvement in England.* London: DH.

DH (2013b) *Health Visiting and School Nursing Programmes: Supporting Implementation of the New Service Model. No.5: Domestic Violence and Abuse – Professional Guidance.* London: DH.

DH (2013c) *Improving Care for People with Dementia.* London: DH. Available at www.gov.uk/government/policies/improving-care-for-people-with-dementia, accessed on 29 May 2013.

DH (2013d) *The Mandate: A Mandate from the Government to the NHS Commissioning Board: April 2013 to March 2015.* London: DH. Available at www.gov.uk/government/publications/the-nhs-mandate, accessed on 20 July 2014.

DH (2013e) *Mental Health Dashboard.* London: DH. Available at www.gov.uk/government/uploads/system/uploads/attachment_data/file/265388/Mental_Health_Dashboard.pdf, accessed on 28 February 2014.

DH (2013f) *NHS Outcomes Framework 2014/15.* London: DH. Available at www.gov.uk/government/publications/nhs-outcomes-framework-2014-to-

2015, accessed on 7 February 2014.

DH (2013g) *Statutory Guidance on Joint Strategic Needs Assessments and Joint Health and Wellbeing Strategies.* London: DH. Available at http://webarchive.nationalarchives. gov.uk/20130805112926/https://s3-eu-west-1.amazonaws.com/media.dh.gov. uk/network/18/files/2013/03/Statutory-Guidance-on-Joint-Strategic-Needs-Assessments-and-Joint-Health-and-Wellbeing-Strategies-March-20131.pdf, accessed on 8 March 2014.

DH (n.d. a) *The General Duties and Powers Relating to Health and Wellbeing Boards.* London: DH. Available at www.gov.uk/government/uploads/system/uploads/ attachment_data/file/144020/General-health-and-wellbeing-board-duties-and-powers.pdf, accessed on 18 April 2014.

DH (n.d. b) *Responsibility Deal.* London: DH. Available at https://responsibilitydeal. dh.gov.uk, accessed on 7 February 2014.

Department of Health Social Security and Public Safety (DHSS&PS) (2011) *Service Framework for Mental Health and Wellbeing.* Belfast: DHSS&PS.

DHSS&PS (2012a) *Health Survey for Northern Ireland.* Belfast: DHSS&PS. Available at www.dhsspsni.gov.uk/health_survey_northern_ireland_-_first_results_from_ the_2011-12_survey.pdf, accessed on 22 February 2014.

DHSS&PS (2012b) *Living with Long Term Conditions.* Belfast: DHSS&PS. Available at www.dhsspsni.gov.uk/living-longterm-conditions.pdf, accessed on 2 December 2013.

DHSS&PS (2014) *Transforming Your Care.* Belfast: DHSS&PS. Available at www. dhsspsni.gov.uk/tyc.htm, accessed on 27 February 2014.

DHSS&PS (n.d.) *Quality Outcomes Framework.* Belfast: DHSS&PS. Available at www. dhsspsni.gov.uk/index/hss/gp_contracts/gp_contract_qof.htm, accessed on 22 February 2014.

Digital Policy Alliance (2013) *Living Independently: Shouldering the Burden of Chronic Disease.* Available at http://dpalliance.org.uk/wp-content/uploads/2013/01/1301_ Telecare-and-Telehealth-Briefing.pdf, accessed on 20 July 2014.

Dobinson, C., MacDonnell, J., Hampson, E., Clipsham, J. and Chow, K. (2003) *Improving the Access and Quality of Public Health Services for Bisexuals.* Toronto: Ontario Public Health Association.

Dockery, A. M., Kendall, G., Li, J., Mahendran, A., Ong, R. and Strazdins, L. (2010) *Housing and Children's Development and Wellbeing: A Scoping Study (AHURI Final Report No. 149).* Melbourne: Australian Housing and Urban Research Institute.

Donabedian, A. (1969) *A Guide to Medical Care Administration Vol 2.* New York, NY: American Public Health Association.

Dorkenoo, E., Morison, L. and Macfarlane, A. (2007) *A Statistical Study to Estimate the Prevalence of Female Genital Mutilation in England and Wales.* London: FORWARD (Foundation for Women's Health, Research and Development).

Druss, B. G., Rosenheck, R. A. and Sledge, W. H. (2000) 'Health and disability costs of depressive illness in a major U.S. corporation.' *American Journal of Psychiatry 157,* 8, 1274–1278.

Duffy, S. (2013) *A Fair Society?* Sheffield: The Centre for Welfare Reform.

Dyer, K. and Teggart, T. (2007) 'Bullying experiences of child and adolescent mental health service-users: A pilot survey.' *Child Care in Practice 13*, 4, 351–365.

Dying Matters (n.d.) *Where do People Want to Die?* Dying Matters. Available at http:// dyingmatters.org/page/frequently-asked-questions, accessed on 30 July 2013.

Ebmeier, S. (2012) *Scottish Parliament Information Centre Briefing: Climate Change and Health in Scotland. Scottish Parliament.* Edinburgh: The Scottish Parliament. Available at www.scottish.parliament.uk/ResearchBriefingsAndFactsheets/S4/ SB_12-26rev.pdf, accessed on 28 April 2013.

Economidoy, E., Klimi, A. and Vivilaki, V. G. (2012) 'Caring for substance abuse pregnant women: The role of the midwife.' *Health Science Journal 6*, 1, 161–169.

Edinburgh Health Inequalities Standing Group (n.d.) *Social Capital, Health and Wellbeing: A Planning and Evaluation Toolkit.* Edinburgh: Edinburgh Health Inequalities Standing Group. Available at www.scdc.org.uk/media/resources/ what-we-do/mtsc/Social%20Capital%20Health%20and%20Wellbeing%20 toolkit.pdf, accessed on 7 August 2013.

Elliott, S. A., Leverton, T. J., Sanjack, M., Turner, H., *et al.* (2000) 'Promoting mental health after childbirth: A controlled trial of primary prevention of postnatal depression.' *The British Journal of Clinical Psychology 39*, 3, 223–241.

Emerson, E. and Baines, S. (2010) *Health Inequalities and People with Learning Disabilities in the UK: 2010.* IHaL. Improving Health and Lives: Learning Disabilities Observatory. Available at www.improvinghealthandlives.org.uk/ uploads/doc/vid_7479_IHaL2010-3HealthInequality2010.pdf, accessed on 19 July 2014.

Entwistle, V. and Cribb, A. (2013) *Enabling People to Live Well: Fresh Thinking about Collaborative Approaches to Care for People with Long-term Conditions.* London: The Health Foundation.

Equality and Human Rights Commission (2010) *Stop and Think: A Critical Review of the Use of Stop and Search Powers in England and Wales.* Equality and Human Rights Commission. Available at www.equalityhumanrights.com/uploaded_files/ raceinbritain/ehrc_stop_and_search_report.pdf, accessed on 11 November 2013.

Ethier, K. A., Kershaw, T. S., Lewis, J. B., Milan, S., Niccolai, L. M. and Ickovics, J. R. (2006) 'Self esteem, emotional distress and sexual behavior among adolescent females: Inter-relationships and temporal effects.' *Journal of Adolescent Health 38*, 3, 268–274.

Evans, O., Singleton, N., Meltzer, H., Stewart, R. and Prince, M. (2003) *The Mental Health of Older People. Report Based on the Analysis of the ONS Survey of Psychiatric Morbidity among Adults in Great Britain Carried Out in 2000 for the Department of Health, the Scottish Executive Health Department and the Welsh Assembly Government.* London: TSO.

Expert Patients Programme (n.d.) *Healthy Lives Equal Healthy Communities – The Social Impact of Self-Management.* London: Expert Patients Programme. Available at www.expertpatients.co.uk/.../EPP%20SROI%20Report_Nov_final_rev2(1).pdf, accessed on 25 July 2014.

Family Mosaic (2013) *Health Begins at Home*. London: Housing LIN (Learning and Improvement Network). Available at www.housinglin.org.uk/pagefinder.cfm?cid=8994, accessed on 19 July 2014.

Family Nurse Partnership National Unit (2012) *The Family Nurse Partnership Programme. Information Leaflet*. London: Department of Health. Available at www.gov.uk/government/uploads/system/uploads/attachment_data/file/216864/The-

Family-Nurse-Partnership-Programme-Information-leaflet.pdf, accessed on 27 August 2013.

Fauth, B., Thompson, M. and Penny, A. (2009) *Associations between Childhood Bereavement and Children's Background, Experiences and Outcomes*. London: National Children's Bureau.

Fear, N. T., Jones, M., Murphy, D., Hull, L., *et al.* (2010) 'What are the consequences of deployment of Iraq and Afghanistan? A cohort study.' *Lancet 375*, 9728, 1783–1797.

Felce, D., Kerr, M. and Hastings, R. P. (2009) 'A general practice-based study of the relationship between indicators of mental illness and challenging behaviour among adults with intellectual disabilities.' *Journal of Intellectual Disability Research 54*, 3, 243–254.

Fellow-Smith, E., Moss-Morris, R., Tylee, A., Fossey, M., Cohen, A. and Nixon, T. (2012) *Investing in Emotional and Psychological Wellbeing for Patients with Long-term Conditions*. London: NHS Confederation.

Ferguson, M., Bannon, E., Hutchinson, B., Clarke, A., *et al.* (2008) *Community Capacity Building*. Belfast: Department of Social Development, Northern Ireland Executive. Available at www.dsdni.gov.uk/vcni-community-capacity-building.pdf, accessed on 25 July 2013.

Fergusson, D. M., Horwood, L. J. and Woodward, L. J. (2001) 'Unemployment and psychosocial adjustment in young adults: Causation or selection?' *Social Science and Medicine 53*, 3, 305–320.

Fernando, S. (2005) 'Multicultural mental health services: Projects for minority ethnic communities in England.' *Transcultural Psychiatry 42*, 3, 420–436.

Fire Service (n.d.) *Free Home Fire Safety Checks*. Available at www.fireservice.co.uk/safety/hfsc, accessed on 6 December 2013.

Flach, C., Leese, M., Heron, J., Evans, J., *et al.* (2011) 'Antenatal domestic violence, maternal mental health and subsequent child behaviour: A cohort study.' *BJOG: An International Journal of Obstetrics and Gynaecology 118*, 11, 1383–1391.

Fletcher, G. J. O. and Kerr, P. S. G. (2010) 'Through the eyes of love: Reality and illusion in intimate relationships.' *Psychological Bulletin 136*, 4, 627–658.

Flint, J. (2010) 'Faith and housing in England: Promoting community cohesion or contributing to urban segregation?' *Journal of Ethnic and Migration Studies. Special Issue: Linking Integration and Residential Segregation 36*, 2, 257–271.

Follett, P. (2011) *An Evidence Base for Population Projections and Long Term Conditions*. York: Yorkshire and Humber Public Health Observatory.

Foot, J. with Hopkins, T. (2010) *A Glass Half-full: How an Asset Approach Can Improve Community Health and Wellbeing.* London: Improvement and Development Agency (IDeA).

Forde, J. and Crook, P. (2013) *HIV Epidemiology in London: 2011 Data.* London: Public Health England.

Foresight Mental Wellbeing and Capital Project (2008) *Mental Capital and Wellbeing: Making the Most of Ourselves in the 21st Century.* London: The Government Office for Science.

Foster, T. (2001) 'Global suicide prevention should focus more on alcohol use disorders.' *British Medical Journal 323*, 817.

Foster, T., Gillespie, K. and McLelland, R. (1997) 'Mental disorders and suicide in Northern Ireland.' *British Journal of Psychiatry 170*, 447–452.

Fox, K. R., Stathi, A., McKenna, J. and Davis, M. D. (2007) 'Physical activity and mental well-being in older people participating in the Better Ageing Project.' *European Journal of Applied Physiology 110*, 5, 591–602.

Faculty of Public Health (FPH) (2008) *Mental Health and Smoking. A Position Statement.* London: FPH.

FPH (2013) *Green Spaces, Mental Health and Wellbeing.* London: Faculty of Public Health. Available at www.fph.org.uk/uploads/bs_great_outdoors.pdf, accessed on 2 January 2014.

Francis, F. and Smith, J. (2002) *Breaking the Circles of Fear.* London: Sainsbury Centre for Mental Health.

French, J., Blair-Stevens, C. and McVey, D. (2010) *Social Marketing and Public Health: Theory and Practice.* Oxford: Oxford University Press.

Friedli, L. (2009) *Mental Health, Resilience and Inequalities. A Report for WHO Europe and the Mental Health Foundation.* London/Copenhagen: Mental Health Foundation and WHO Europe.

Friedli, L. (2012) '"What we've tried, hasn't worked": The politics of assets based public health.' *Critical Public Health.* Available at http://dx.doi.org/10.1080/09581596.20 12.748882, accessed on 20 February 2014.

Friedli, L., Jackson, C., Abernethy, H. and Stansfield, J. (2009) *Social Prescribing for Mental Health – A Guide to Commissioning and Delivery.* Hyde: CSIP (Care Services Improvement Partnership).

Friedman, M. S., Marshal, M. P., Guadamuz, T. E., Wei, C., *et al.* (2011) 'A meta-analysis of disparities in childhood sexual abuse, parental physical abuse, and peer victimization among sexual minority and sexual nonminority individuals.' *American Journal of Public Health 101*, 8, 1481–1494.

Friguls, B., Jova, S., Garcia-Algar, O., Pallas, C. R., Vall, O. and Pichini, S. (2010) 'A comprehensive review of assay methods to determine drugs in breast milk and the safety of breastfeeding when taking drugs.' *Bioanalytical Chemistry 397*, 3, 1157–1179.

Galtung, J. and Jacobsen, C. G. (2000) *Searching for Peace: The Road to TRANSCEND.* London: Pluto Press.

Garner, S. and Bhattacharyya, G. (2011) *Poverty, Ethnicity and Place.* York: Joseph Rowntree Foundation.

Gillborn, D. (2008) 'Coincidence or conspiracy? Whiteness, policy and the persistence of the black/white achievement gap.' *Educational Review 60,* 3, 229–248.

Glasgow Centre for Population Health (2011) *Asset Based Approach for Health Improvement: Redressing the Balance.* Glasgow: Glasgow Centre for Population Health.

Glassman, P. (2013) *Health Literacy.* Bethesda, Maryland: National Network of Libraries of Medicine. Available at http://nnlm.gov/outreach/consumer/hlthlit.html, accessed on 26 August 2013.

Goodwin, N., Dixon, A., Poole, T. and Raleigh, V. (2011) *Improving the Quality of Care in General Practice.* London: The King's Fund.

Goodwin, R. D., Sourander, A., Duarte, C. S., Niemelä, S., *et al.* (2009) 'Do mental health problems in childhood predict chronic physical conditions among males in early adulthood? Evidence from a community-based prospective study.' *Psychological Medicine 39,* 2, 301–311.

Gov.UK (2014) *Workplace Bullying and Harassment.* Gov.UK. Available at www.gov.uk/workplace-bullying-and-harassment, accessed on 15 April 2014.

Gov.UK (n.d.) *Police Powers to Stop and Search: Your Rights.* Gov.UK. Available at www.gov.uk/police-powers-to-stop-and-search-your-rights, accessed on 21 November 2013.

Graham, H. (2010) 'Where is the future in public health?' *Milbank Quarterly 88,* 2, 149–168.

Graham, H. (2012) 'Ensuring the health of future populations.' *BMJ 2012.345e7573.*

Grahn, P. and Stigsdotter, U. K. (2010) 'The relation between perceived sensory dimensions of urban green space and stress restoration.' *Landscape and Urban Planning 90,* 3–4, 264–275.

Gray, S., Carmichael, L., Barton, H., Mytton, J., Lease, H. and Joynt, J. (2011) 'The effectiveness of health appraisal processes currently in addressing health and wellbeing during spatial plan appraisal: A systematic review.' *BMC Public Health 11,* 889. Available at www.biomedcentral.com/1471-2458/11/889, accessed on 24 June 2014.

Green, H., McGinnity, A., Meltzer, H., Ford, T. and Goodman, R. (2005) *Mental Health of Children and Young People in Great Britain.* Basingstoke: Palgrave Macmillan.

Greene, R., Pugh, R. and Roberts, D. (2008) *Black and Minority Ethnic Parents with Mental Health Problems and their Children. Research Briefing 29.* London: Social Care Institute for Excellence.

Gregoire, A. and Mayers, A. (2006) *Rural Mental Health Research Project. Final Report.* Southampton: National Mental Health Partnership.

Griffin, J. (2010) *The Lonely Society?* London: Mental Health Foundation.

Grossman, R. and Scala, K. (1993) *Health Promotion and Organizational Development: Developing Settings for Health.* Vienna: WHO Europe.

Gunnell, D., Peters, T., Kammerling, M. and Brooks, J. (1995) 'The relationship between parasuicide, suicide, psychiatric admissions and socioeconomic deprivation.' *British Medical Journal 311*, 226–230.

Halliwell, E. (2005) *Up and Running: Exercise Therapy and the Treatment of Mild or Moderate Depression in Primary Care.* London: Mental Health Foundation.

Halpern, D. S. (1993) 'Minorities and mental health.' *Social Science and Medicine 36*, 597–607.

Hamer, L., Killoran, A., Macknight, A. and Falce, C. (2006) *Health Equity Audit – Learning from Practice Briefing.* London: National Institute for Health and Clinical Excellence.

Hammond, C. and Feinstein, L. (2006) *Are Those who Flourished at School Healthier Adults? What Role for Adult Education? Wider Benefits of Learning Research Report No. 17.* Missoula, Montana: Center for Research on the Wider Benefits of Learning. Available at www.learningbenefits.net/Publications/ResReps/ResRep17.pdf, accessed on 2 January 2013.

Hampton, C. and Heaven, C. (2013) *Understanding and Describing the Community. Lawrence, Kansas: Community Tool Box,* University of Kansas. Available at http://ctb.ku.edu, accessed on 24 June 2014.

Hanley, O. (2013) 'Co-production in Scotland – A Network for Change.' In E. Loeffler, G. Power, T. Bovaird and F. Hine-Hughes (eds) *Co-production of Health and Wellbeing in Scotland.* Birmingham: Governance International.

Hanlon, P., Carlisle, S., Lyon, A., Hannah, M. and Reilly, D. (2013) *The Future Public Health: An Integrative Framework.* Glasgow: AfterNow. Available at http://afternow.co.uk/sites/default/files/The%20future%20public%20health%20-%20an%20integrative%20framework.pdf, accessed on 28 October 2013.

Harries, B. and Richardson, L. (2009) 'Citizen Aspirations: Women, Ethnicity and Housing.' In C. Durose, S. Greasley and L. Richardson (eds) *Changing Local Governance, Changing Citizens.* Bristol: Policy Press.

Harris-Roxas, B., Viliani, F., Bond, A., Cave, B., *et al.* (2012) 'Health impact assessment: The state of the art.' *Impact Assessment and Project Appraisal 30*, 1, 43–52.

Harriss, K. and Salway, S. (2008) *Long-term Ill Health, Poverty and Ethnicity.* London: Race Equality Foundation.

Harvey, S. B., Hotopf, M., Øverland, S. and Mykletun, A. (2010) 'Physical activity and common mental disorders.' *British Journal of Psychiatry 197*, 357–364.

Hawe, P., King, L., Noort, M., Jordens, C. and Lloyd, B. (2000) *Indicators to Help with Capacity Building in Health Promotion.* Sydney: NSW Health. Available at www.health.nsw.gov.au/pubs/2000/pdf/capbuild.pdf, accessed on 30 September 2013.

Hawes, P., Webster, C. and Sheill, A. (2004) 'A glossary of terms for navigating the field of social network analysis.' *Journal of Epidemiology and Community Health 58*, 971–975.

Hawton, A., Green, C., Dickens, A. P., Richards, S. H., *et al.* (2011) 'The impact of social isolation on the health status and health-related quality of life of older people.' *Quality of Life Research 20*, 57–67.

Hawton, K. and Haw, C. (2013) 'Economic recession and suicide.' *British Medical Journal 2013;347f5612.*

Health Behaviour in School-aged Children (HBSC) (2011) *England National Report.* Hatfield: University of Hertfordshire.

Health Education Authority (HEA) (1999) *Black and Minority Ethnic Groups and Tobacco Use in England.* London: HEA.

Health Impact Assessment (HIA) Gateway (2013) Birmingham: Association of Public Health Observatories. Available at www.apho.org.uk/default.aspx?QN=P_HIA, accessed on 19 August 2013.

Health Protection Agency (2012) *STI Data from Genitourinary Medicine (GUM) Clinics.* London: Health Protection Agency.

Heath, A. and Khan, O. (2012) *Ethnic Minority British Election Study – Key Findings.* London: Runnymede Trust. Available at www.runnymedetrust.org/uploads/EMBESbriefingFINALx.pdf, accessed on 18 November 2013.

Hex, N. and Tatlock, S. (2011) *Altogether Better Social Return on Investment Case Studies. A Report Commissioned by Altogether Better Learning Network, Yorkshire and Humber Public Health Observatory.* York: York Health Economics Consortium.

Hicks, S. (2013) *Differences in Well-being by Ethnicity.* London: Office for National Statistics (ONS).

Hiday, V. A. (2006) 'Putting community risk in perspective: A look at correlations, causes and controls.' *International Journal of Law and Psychiatry 29,* 316–331.

Higgins, V. and Dale, A. (2010) *Ethnic Differences in Physical Activity, Diet and Obesity.* Manchester: University of Manchester.

HM Government (2008) *The Nation's Commitment: Cross-government support to our Armed Forces, their families and veterans CM 7424.* London: TSO, available at www.gov.uk/government/publications, accessed 23 September 2014.

HM Government (2010a) *Drug Strategy 2010. Reducing Demand, Restricting Supply, Building Recovery: Supporting People to Live a Drug Free Life.* London: HM Government. Available at www.gov.uk/government/uploads/system/uploads/attachment_data/file/118336/drug-strategy-2010.pdf, accessed on 7 February 2014.

HM Government (2010b) *Pursue Prevent Protect Prepare: The United Kingdom's Strategy for Countering International Terrorism. Annual Report.* Norwich/London: TSO.

HM Government (2012a) *Caring for Our Future: Reforming Care and Support CM 8378.* London: TSO.

HM Government (2012b) *Challenge it, Report it, Stop it: The Government's Plan to Tackle Hate Crime.* London: HM Government.

HM Government (2012c) *The Government's Alcohol Strategy CM8336.* Norwich: TSO.

HM Government and DH (2011) *No Health without Mental Health: A Cross-government Mental Health Outcomes Strategy for People of All Ages. Gateway Reference 14679.* London: DH.

HM Government and DH (2012) *Preventing Suicide in England: A Cross-government Outcomes Strategy to Save Lives.* London: DH.

Her Majesty's Inspectorate of Prisons (HMIP) (2012) *Expectations: Criteria for Assessing the Treatment of Prisoners and Conditions in Prisons.* London: HMIP. Available at www.justice.gov.uk/downloads/about/hmipris/adult-expectations-2012.pdf, accessed on 20 November 2013.

HM Treasury (2006) *Stern Review on the Economics of Climate Change.* London: HM Treasury.

Hoare, J. and Moon, D. (2010) *Drug Misuse Declared: Findings from the 2009/10 British Crime Survey England and Wales.* London: Home Office.

Holley, U. A. (2007) 'Social isolation: A practical guide for nurses assisting clients with chronic illness.' *Rehabilitation Nursing 32*, 2, 51–58.

Home Office (2012) *Putting Victims First: More Effective Responses to Anti-social Behaviour.* Norwich: TSO.

Home Office (2013a) *A New Approach to Fighting Crime.* London: Home Office. Available at www.gov.uk/government/uploads/system/uploads/attachment_data/file/97825/new-approach-fighting-crime.pdf, accessed on 20 April 2013.

Home Office (2013b) *Call to End Violence Against Women and Girls: Action Plan.* London: Home Office.

Hoong Sin, C., Hedges, A., Cook, C., Mguni, N. and Comber, N. (2009) *Disabled People's Experiences of Targeted Violence and Hostility.* London: Office for Public Management/Equality and Human Rights Commission.

Hope, S., Power, C. and Rodgers, B. (1999) 'Does financial hardship account for elevated psychological distress in lone mothers?' *Social Science and Medicine 49*, 1637–1649.

Hopton, J. L. and Hunt, S. M. (1996) 'Housing conditions and mental health in a disadvantaged area in Scotland.' *Journal of Epidemiology and Community Health 50*, 56–61.

Horvitz-Lennon, M., Normand, S.-L. T., Gaccione, P. and Frank, R. G. (2001) 'Partial versus full hospitalization for adults in psychiatric distress: A systematic review of the published literature (1957–1997).' *American Journal of Psychiatry 158*, 676–685.

Hothi, M., with Bacon, N., Brophy, M. and Mulgan, G. (2008) *Neighbourliness + Empowerment = Wellbeing. Is there a Formula for Happy Communities?* London: LSE (London School of Economics). Available at www.lse.ac.uk/intranet/LSEServices/ERD/pressAndInformationOffice/PDF/NeighbourlinessEmpowermentWellbeing.pdf, accessed on 18 November 2013.

House of Lords and House of Commons Joint Committee (2012–2013) *Care and Support Bill. Draft Care and Support Bill Report.* London: TSO.

Howard, L. M. (2005) 'Fertility and pregnancy in women with psychotic disorders.' *European Journal of Obstetrics, Gynaecology and Reproductive Biology 119*, 1, 3–10.

Howarth, G. (2011) *Veterans' ('Ex-Military') Health Needs Assessment for Kent and Medway.* Kent/Medway: NHS Kent and Medway.

Health and Social Care Information Centre (HSCIC) (2013a) *Disease Prevalence, Quality and Outcomes Framework, April 2012–March 2013, England.* Leeds: HSCIC. Available at www.hscic.gov.uk/catalogue/PUB12262, accessed on 19 March 2014.

HSCIC (2013b) *Health Survey for England 2012. Health, Social Care and Lifestyles: Summary of Key Findings*. Leeds: HSCIC.

HSCIC (n.d. a) *Mental Health Minimum Data Set*. Leeds: HSCIC. Available at www.hscic.gov.uk/mhmds, accessed on 12 February 2014.

HSCIC (n.d. b) *Quality and Outcomes Framework*. Leeds: HSCIC. Available at www.hscic.gov.uk/qof, accessed on 12 February 2014.

Hudson, M., Netto, G., Sosenko, F., Noon, M., *et al.* (2013) *In-Work Poverty, Ethnicity and Workplace Cultures*. York: Joseph Rowntree Foundation.

Hughes, L. (2006) *Closing the Gap. A Capability Framework for Working Effectively with People with Combined Mental Health and Substance Use Problems (Dual Diagnosis)*. Lincoln: Centre for Clinical and Academic Workforce Innovation, University of Lincoln.

Hunter, D. J. (2003) *Public Health Policy*. Cambridge, UK: Polity Press.

Hurcombe, R., Bayley, M. and Goodman, A. (2010) *Ethnicity and Alcohol: A Review of the UK Literature*. York: Joseph Rowntree Foundation.

Husband, H., Carr, P. and Jepson, W. (2010) *Guidance on Involving Adult NHS Service Users and Carers*. Llanharan: National Leadership and Innovation Agency for Healthcare.

Improving Access to Psychological Therapies (IAPT) (n.d.). *Models of Care*. Available at www.iapt.nhs.uk, accessed on 24 July 2014.

Institute of Alcohol Studies (IAS) (2007) *Alcohol and Mental Health. IAS Factsheet*. St Ives: Institute of Alcohol Studies.

IAS (2010) *Alcohol and the Elderly. IAS Factsheet*. St Ives: Institute of Alcohol Studies.

International Conflict Research Institute (INCORE) & The Community Foundation for Northern Ireland (2006, updated 2010) *Guide to Peacebuilding in Northern Ireland*. Londonderry: University of Ulster. Available at www.incore.ulst.ac.uk/services/cds/newcfni/intervention, accessed on 1 February 2014.

Inglis, J. (2012) *Guide to Commissioning for Maximum Value*. London: Local Government Association.

Institute of Race Relations (n.d.) *Poverty, Inequality, Employment and Health*. London: Institute of Race Relations. Available at www.irr.org.uk/research/statistics/poverty, accessed on 11 November 2013.

Ipsos MORI (2011) *Long Term Health Conditions 2011. Research Study Conducted for the Department of Health*. Leeds: Long Term Conditions, DH.

Institute for Research and Innovation in Social Services (IRISS) (2010) *Improving Support for Black and Minority Ethnic (BME) Carers*. Glasgow: IRISS. Available at www.iriss.org.uk/sites/default/files/iriss-insight-7.pdf, accessed on 21 November 2013.

ISD (Information Services Division) Scotland (n.d.) *Quality & Outcomes Framework (QOF)*. Edinburgh and Glasgow: ISD Scotland. Available at www.isdscotland.org/Health-Topics/General-Practice/Quality-And-Outcomes-Framework, accessed on 20 February 2014.

Iverson, A. C., van Staden, L., Hughes, J. H., Hull, L., *et al.* (2009) 'The prevalence of common mental disorders and PTSD in the UK military: Using data from a clinical interview-based study.' *BME Psychiatry 9*, 68.

James, L., Brody, D. and Hamilton, Z. (2013) 'Risk factors for domestic violence during pregnancy: A meta-analytic review.' *Violence and Victims 28*, 3, 359–380.

Jansson, K. (2007) *British Crime Survey – Measuring Crime for 25 Years.* Available at http://webarchive.nationalarchives.gov.uk/20110218135832/rds.homeoffice.gov.uk/rds/pdfs07/bcs25.pdf, accessed on 6 December 2013.

Joint Commissioning Panel for Mental Health (JCPMH) (2013) *Guidance for Commissioning Public Mental Health Services.* JCPMH. Available at www.jcpmh.info/wp-content/uploads/jcpmh-publicmentalhealth-guide.pdf, accessed on 19 July 2014.

Jewkes, R. K. and Murcott, A. (1998) 'Community representatives: Representing the "community"?' *Social Science and Medicine 6*, 843–858.

Johnsen, S., Jones, A. and Rugg, J. (2008) *The Experience of Homeless Ex-service Personnel in London.* York: Centre for Housing Policy, University of York.

Johnson, N. (2011) *Assessing the Economic and Social Cost of Suicide and Attempted Suicide.* Durham: North East Mental Health Development Unit (NEMHDU). Available at www.nemhdu.org.uk/silo/files/economic-costs-of-suicide-march-2011.pdf, accessed on 24 February 2014.

Johnson, N. and Johnson, P. (2011) *Fighting Fit in the North East.* Durham: North East Mental Health Development Unit.

Johnson, N. and Ross, L. (2011) *Social Prescribing within the North East: Current Programmes and Challenges for the Future.* Durham: North East Mental Health Development Unit.

Johnson, R., Griffiths, C. and Nottingham, T. (2006) *At Home? Mental Health Issues Arising in Social Housing.* London: National Institute for Mental Health in England.

Joint Committee on Human Rights (2004) *Deaths in Custody: Third Report of Session 2004– 05.* London: House of Lords/House of Commons Justice. Available at www.publications.parliament.uk/pa/jt200405/jtselect/jtrights/15/1502.htm, accessed on 18 July 2014.

Joloza, T., Evans, J., O'Brien, R. and Potter-Collins, A. (2010) *Measuring Sexual Identity: An Evaluation Report.* Newport: Office for National Statistics.

Jones, A. (2011) *Brighton and Hove Youth Service Needs Assessment.* Brighton and Hove: Brighton and Hove NHS/Brighton and Hove City Council.

Jones, A., Jeyasingham, D. and Rajasooriya, S. (2002) *The Strengths and Needs of Black Families in which Young People have Caring Responsibilities.* York: Joseph Rowntree Foundation.

Jones, I. and Craddock, N. (2005) 'Bipolar disorder and childbirth: The importance of recognising risk.' *British Journal of Psychiatry 186*, 452–454.

Kabat-Zinn, J. (2012) *Mindfulness for Beginners.* Louisville, Colorado: Sounds True, Inc.

Kammerling, M. and O'Connor, S. (1993) 'Unemployment rate as predictor of rate of psychiatric admission.' *British Medical Journal 307*, 1536–1539.

Kapur, N., While, D., Blatchley, N., Bray, I. and Harrison, K. (2009) 'Suicide after leaving the UK Armed Forces – A cohort study.' *PLoS Med 6, 3. doi: 10.1371/journal. pmed.1000026.* Available at www.plosmedicine.org/article/info:doi/10.1371/journal.pmed.1000026, accessed on 12 January 2013.

Katz, I., La Placa, V. and Hunter, S. (2007) *Barriers to Inclusion and Successful Engagement of Parents in Mainstream Services.* York: Joseph Rowntree Foundation.

Kawachi, I., Kennedy, B. P. and Lochner, K. (1997) 'Long live community: Social capital as public health.' *The American Prospect 8*, 35 (November–December), 56–59.

Kearns, A., Whitley, E., Bond, L., Egan, M. and Tannahill, C. (2013) 'The psychosocial pathway to mental well-being at the local level: Investigating the effects of perceived relative position in a deprived area context.' *Journal of Epidemiology and Community Health 67*, 87–94.

Keating, F., Robertson, D., McCulloch, A. and Francis, A. (2002) *Breaking the Circles of Fear: A Review of the Relationship between Mental Health Services and African and Caribbean Communities.* London: Sainsbury Centre for Mental Health.

Kenagy, G. P. (2005) 'Transgender health: Findings from two needs assessment studies in Philadelphia.' *Health & Social Work 31*, 1, 19–26.

Kennedy, R. and Phillips, J. (2011) 'Social Return on Investment (SROI): A case study with an expert patient programme.' *SelfCare, The Journal of Consumer-led Health 2*, 1, 10–20.

Kent, M., Davis, M. C. and Reich, J. W. (eds) (2014) *The Resilience Handbook.* New York, NY/Hove: Routledge.

Kim, Y. S., Park, Y. S., Allegrante, J. P., Marks, R., *et al.* (2012) 'Relationship between physical activity and general mental health.' *Preventative Medicine 55*, 5, 458–463.

King, C., Fulford, B., Williamson, T., Dhillon, K. and Vasiliou-Theodore, C. (2009) *Model Values: Race, Values and Models in Mental Health.* London: Mental Health Foundation.

Kleinman, A. (2012) 'Culture, bereavement and psychiatry.' *The Lancet 379*, 9816, 608–609.

Knifton, L., Gervais, M., Newbigging, K., Mirza, N., *et al.* (2010) 'Community conversation:

Addressing mental health stigma with ethnic minority communities.' *Social Psychiatry and Psychiatric Epidemiology 45*, 4, 497–504.

Kosunen, E., Kaltiala-Heino, R., Rimpelä, M. and Laippala, P. (2003) 'Risk-taking sexual behaviour and self-reported depression in middle adolescence – A school-based survey.' *Child Care and Health Development 29*, 5, 337–344.

Kuo, F. and Sullivan, W. C. (2001) 'Environment and crime in the inner city: Does vegetation reduce crime?' *Environment and Behaviour 33*, 3, 343–346.

Kuosmanen, L., Vuorilehto, M., Kumpuniemi, S. and Melartin, T. (2010) 'Post-natal depression screening and treatment in maternity and child health clinics.' *Journal of Psychiatric and Mental Health Nursing 17*, 6, 554–557.

Kurtz, Z. and Street, C. (2006) 'Mental health services for young people from black and minority ethnic backgrounds: The current challenge.' *Journal of Children's Services 1*, 3, 40–49.

Lacey, K. K., McPherson, M. D., Samual, P. S., Sears, K. P. and Head, D. (2013) 'The impact of different types of intimate partner violence on the mental and physical health of women in different ethnic groups.' *Journal of Interpersonal Violence 28*, 2, 359–385.

LaRocca, R., Yost, J., Ciliska, D. and Dobbins, M. (2013) '*The effectiveness of knowledge translation and exchange strategies used in public health.*' Paper presented at *FUSE Conference*, Holland. Available at: www.tilburguniversity.edu/migration-temp/tranzo/hollandfuseconference/abstracts, accessed on 25 June 2014.

Last, J. M. (ed.) (1995) *A Dictionary of Epidemiology, Third Edition.* New York, NY: Oxford University Press.

Lau, A., Black, A. and Sturdy, V. (2008) *Delivering Race Equality: Improving BME Outcomes in Education and Employment. A London Survey of Early Intervention in Psychosis Teams and Links with the Further Education System.* Leicester: National Institute of Adult Continuing Education.

Learmonth, A. (2013) 'Knowledge exchange through public health commissioning to improve health and reduce inequalities in Gateshead 2008–2012.' *FUSE Conference: How to Get Practice into Science*, Holland. Available at www.tilburguniversity.edu/upload/a2abfe49-a926-4c8a-abf6-5e8c37b45efd_parallelsession3.pdf, accessed on 17 April 2014.

Learmonth, A. and Curtis, S. (2012) *Place Making for Health: Health Impact Assessment as a Tool for System Change to Address Inequalities in Health at a Local Level.* Birmingham: HIA Gateway. Available at www.apho.org.uk/resource/browse.aspx?RID=121323, accessed on 11 March 2013.

Lee, J. K., Jackson, H. J., Pattison, P. and Ward, T. (2002) 'Developmental risk factors for sexual offending.' *Child Abuse and Neglect 26*, 1, 73–92.

Leeds City Council (2013) *Inequality to Inclusion.* Leeds: Leeds City Council. Available at www.leeds.gov.uk/docs/LEH%2007%20Inequality%20to%20inclusion.pdf, accessed on 21 November 2013.

Lees, S. (2000) 'Marital Rape and Marital Murder.' In J. Hanmer and N. Itzin (eds) *Home Truths about Domestic Violence: Feminist Influences on Policy and Practice: A Reader.* London: Routledge.

Lehrer, J. A., Shrier, L. A., Gortmaker, S. and Buka, S. (2006) 'Depressive symptoms as a longitudinal predictor of sexual risk behaviors among US middle and high school students.' *Pediatrics 118*, 1, 189–200.

Lewis, G. and Drife, J. (2004) *Why Mothers Die 2000–2002: The Sixth Report of Confidential Enquiries into Maternal Death in the United Kingdom.* London: Confidential Enquiry into Maternal and Child Health (CEMACH)/Royal College of Obstetricians and Gynaecologists.

Lewis, M. (2013) 'Foreword.' In M. Parsonage (ed.) *Welfare Advice for People Who Use Mental Health Services: Developing the Business Case.* London: Centre for Mental Health.

Liddell, C. and Morris, C. (2010) 'Fuel poverty and human health: A review of recent evidence.' *Energy Policy 38*, 6, 2987–2997.

Lobel, M., Dunkel-Schetter, C. and Scrimshaw, S. C. (1992) 'Prenatal maternal stress and prematurity: A prospective study of socio-economically disadvantaged women.' *Health Psychology 11*, 32–40.

London's Poverty Profile (2013) *Ethnicity, Low Income and Work.* London: Trust for London and New Policy Institute. Available at www.londonspovertyprofile.org.uk/indicators/topics/ethnicity-low-income-and-work, accessed on 21 November 2013.

Lou, H. C., Hansen, D., Nordentoft, M., Pryds, O., *et al.* (1994) 'Prenatal stressors of human life affect fetal brain development.' *Developmental Medicine and Child Neurology 36*, 826–832.

Lovestone, S. and Kumar, R. (1993) 'Postnatal psychiatric illness: The impact on partners.' *The British Journal of Psychiatry 163*, 210–216.

Low, N., Sterne, J. A. and Barlow, D. (2001) 'Inequalities in rates of gonorrhoea and chlamydia between black ethnic groups in south east London: Cross sectional study.' *Sexually Transmitted Infections 77*, 1, 15–20.

Low Pay Commission (2013) *National Minimum Wage: Low Pay Commission Report 2013. Cm 8565.* London: TSO.

Luanaigh, C. O. and Lawlor, B. A. (2008) 'Loneliness and the health of older people.' *International Journal of Geriatric Psychiatry 23*, 12, 1213–1221.

Lundin, A. and Hemmingsson, T. (2009) 'Unemployment and suicide.' *The Lancet 374*, 9686, 270–271.

Lynch, J. W., Kaplan, G. A. and Shema, S. J. (1997) 'Cumulative impact of sustained economic hardship on physical, cognitive, psychological and social functioning.' *New England Journal of Medicine 337*, 1889–1895.

Mackereth, C. J. (2009) *Mental Health Needs Assessment of the Population of NHS South of Tyne and Wear: Gateshead, South Tyneside and Sunderland.* Sunderland: NHS South of Tyne and Wear.

Mackereth, C. J. and Appleton, J. (2008) 'Social networks and health inequalities – the evidence for working with disadvantaged groups.' *Community Practitioner 81*, 8, 23–26.

Mandiberg, J. M. (2012) 'Commentary. The failure of social inclusion: An alternative approach through community development.' *Psychiatric Services 63*, 5, 458–460.

Manning, C. and White, P. D. (1995) 'Attitudes of employers to the mentally ill.' *The Psychiatrist 19*, 541–543.

Markkanen, S., with Clarke, A., Fenton, A., Holmans, A., Monk, S. and Whitehead, C. (2008) *Understanding Demographic, Special and Economic Impacts on Future Affordable Housing Demand. Paper Five – BME Housing Needs and Aspirations.* Cambridge, UK: Cambridge Centre for Housing and Planning Design.

Marmot, M. (2010a) *Fair Society, Fair Lives (The Marmot Review). Executive Summary.* London: The Marmot Review.

Marmot, M. (2010b) *Fair Society, Fair Lives (The Marmot Review). Strategic Review of Health Inequalities in England post 2010.* London: Department of Health.

Martin, K. and Hart, R. (2011) *'Trying to Get By': Consulting with Children and Young People on Child Poverty.* London: Office of the Children's Commissioner.

Mass, J., Verheij, R. A., Groenewegen, P. P., de Vries, S. and Speeuwenbergy, P. (2006) 'Green space, urbanity, and health: How strong is the relation?' *Journal of Epidemiology and Community Health 60*, 587–592.

May, T., Gyateng, T. and Bateman, T. (2009) *Exploring the Needs of Young Black and Minority Ethnic Offenders and the Provision of Targeted Interventions.* London: Criminal Policy Research, King's College London.

Mayo Clinic (2014) *Nutrition and Healthy Eating.* Rochester, Minnesota: Mayo Clinic. Available at www.mayoclinic.org/healthy-living/nutrition-and-healthy-eating/in-depth/food-and-nutrition/art-20048294, accessed on 16 April 2014.

Mays, V. M. and Cochran, S. D. (2001) 'Mental health correlates of perceived discrimination among lesbian, gay, and bisexual adults in the United States.' *American Journal of Public Health 91*, 11, 1869–1876.

McCabe, A., Gilchrist, A., Harris, K., Afridi, A. and Kyprianou, P. (2013) *Making the Links: Poverty, Ethnicity and Social Networks.* York: Joseph Rowntree Foundation.

McCarthy, M. I. and Zeggini, E. (2009) 'Genome-wide association studies in type 2 diabetes.' *Current Diabetes Reports 9*, 164–171.

McConkey, R., Nixon, T., Donaghy, E. and Mulhern, C. (2004) 'The characteristics of children with a disability looked after away from home and their future service needs.' *British Journal of Social Work 34*, 4, 561–576.

McCrone, P., Dhansairi, S., Patel, A., Knapp, M. and Lawton-Smith, S. (2008) *Paying the Price.* London: King's Fund.

McDaid, L. M., Ross, G. and Young, I. (2012) *Men, Deprivation and Sexual Health: Scoping Review. Occasional Paper No. 22.* Glasgow: University of Glasgow MRC (Medical Research Council)/CSO (Chief Scientist Office) Social and Public Health Sciences Unit.

McLeod, S. A. (2007) *John Bowlby: Maternal Deprivation Theory. Simply Psychology.* Available at www.simplypsychology.org/bowlby.html, accessed on 28 July 2013.

McNamee, H. (2006) *Out on Your Own: An Examination of the Mental Health of Young Same-sex Attracted Men.* Belfast: The Rainbow Project.

Mead, G. E., Morley, W., Campbell, P., Greig, C. A., McMurdo, M. and Lawlor, D. A. (2009) *Exercise for Depression. Cochrane Database Systematic Review, 3:CD004366.* Available at www.ncbi.nlm.nih.gov/pubmed/18843656, accessed on 22 June 2012.

Meltzer, H., Doos, L., Vostanis, P., Ford, T. and Goodman, R. (2009) 'The mental health of children who witness domestic violence.' *Child and Family Social Work 14*, 4, 491–501.

Meltzer, H., Gatward, R., Goodman, R. and Ford, T. (2000) *Mental Health of Children and Adolescents in Great Britain.* London: TSO.

Meltzer, H., Gill, B. and Petticrew, M. (1995) *The Prevalence of Psychiatric Morbidity among Adults Living in Private Households.* London: HMSO.

Mencap (2007) *Bullying Wrecks Lives: The Experiences of Children and Young People with a Learning Disability.* London: Mencap.

Menezes, P. R., Johnson, S., Thornicroft, G., Marshall, J., *et al.* (1996) 'Drug and alcohol problems amongst individuals with severe mental illness in South London.' *British Journal of Psychiatry 168*, 612–619.

Mental Health Foundation (2002) *The Mental Health Needs of Homeless Children and Young People.* London: Mental Health Foundation.

Mental Health Foundation (2007) *The Fundamental Facts.* London: Mental Health Foundation.

Mental Health Foundation (2010a) *Executive Briefing: The Mental Health of Veterans.* London: Mental Health Foundation.

Mental Health Foundation (2010b) *Grouchy Old Men: A Brief Guide to Help Develop Services that Engage Isolated Older Men and Promote Good Mental Health and Well Being.* London: Mental Health Foundation.

Mental Health Foundation (2010c) *The Lonely Society.* London: Mental Health Foundation.

Mental Health Foundation (2011) *How to Look After Your Mental Health in Later Life.* London: Mental Health Foundation.

Mental Health Foundation (2012) *Mid-life Women and Mental Health.* London: Mental Health Foundation.

Mental Health Foundation (n.d. a) *Black and Minority Ethnic Communities.* London: Mental Health Foundation. Available at www.mentalhealth.org.uk/help-information/mental-health-a-z/B/BME-communities, accessed on 25 June 2014.

Mental Health Foundation (n.d. b) *Mental Health Statistics: Men and Women.* London: Mental Health Foundation. Available at www.mentalhealth.org.uk/help-information/mental-health-statistics/men-women, accessed on 29 May 2013.

Mental Health Foundation (n.d. c) *Recovery.* London: Mental Health Foundation. Available at www.mentalhealth.org.uk/help-information/mental-health-a-z/R/recovery, accessed on 18 March 2014.

Mental Health Reporting (2013) *Facts about Mental Illness and Violence.* Warwick: School of Social Work, The University of Warwick. Available at http://depts.washington.edu/mhreport/facts_violence.php, accessed on 9 March 2013.

Mental Health (Wales) Measure (2010) Cardiff: National Assembly for Wales.

Mepham, S. (2010) 'Disabled children: The right to feel safe.' *Child Care in Practice 16,* 1, 19–34.

Meyer, I. H. (2003) 'Prejudice, social stress and mental health in lesbian, gay and bisexual populations: Conceptual issues and research evidence.' *Psychological Bulletin 129,* 674–697.

Mezey, G. (1997) 'Domestic Violence in Pregnancy.' In S. Bewley, J. Friend and G. Mezey (eds) *Violence against Women.* London: Royal College of Obstetricians and Gynaecologists.

Michael, J. (2008) *Healthcare for All. Report of the Independent Inquiry into Access to Healthcare for People with Learning Disabilities.* Department of Health. Available at http://webarchive.nationalarchives.gov.uk/20130107105354/http:/www.dh.gov.uk/en/Publicationsandstatistics/Publications/PublicationsPolicyAndGuidance/DH_099255, accessed on 18 July 2014.

Michaelson, J., Abdullah, S., Steuer, N., Thompson, S. and Marks, N. (2009) *National Accounts of Well-being – Bringing Real Wealth onto the Balance Sheet.* London: New Economics Foundation.

Michalak, E. E., Yatham, L. N., Maxwell, V., Hale, S. and Lam, R. W. (2007) 'The impact of bipolar disorder upon work functioning: A qualitative analysis.' *Bipolar Disorders 9*, 1–2, 126.

Miles, N., Tully, J., Hudson, F., Queau, K. and Rotheroe, N. (2005) *Social Capital and Economic Development in the North East of England: Promoting Economic Inclusion through Community Based Programmes and Projects.* Stockton-on-Tees: University of Durham.

Mills, H. (2003) *Meeting the Needs of Black and Minority Ethnic Young Carers: A Literature Review and Research Study for the Willow Young Carers Service.* London: Barnardo's Policy, Research and Influencing Unit.

Mind (2013) *Making Sense of Ecotherapy.* London and Cardiff: Mind.

Mind (n.d. a) *About Debt.* London and Cardiff: Mind. Available at www.mind.org.uk/information-support/guides-to-support-and-services/debt-and-mental-health/about-debt/?o=6845, accessed on 18 January 2014.

Mind (n.d. b) *Housing and Mental Health.* London and Cardiff: Mind. Available at www.mind.org.uk/information-support/guides-to-support-and-services/housing, accessed on 18 January 2014.

Mironski, M. (2010) *Sexual Health Needs Assessment: Black and Minority Ethnic.* Hull and East Riding of Yorkshire: Network, Hull and East Riding Sexual and Reproductive Healthcare Partnership.

Mirrlees-Black, C. (1999) *Domestic Violence: Findings from a New British Crime Survey Self Completion Questionnaire. Home Office Research Study 191.* London: Home Office.

Mitchell, M., Howarth, C., Kotecha, M. and Creegan, C. (2008) *Sexual Orientation Research Review 2008.* Manchester: Equality and Human Rights Commission.

Ministry of Justice (MoJ) (2010) *Statistics on Women and the Criminal Justice System.* London: MoJ. Available at www.justice.gov.uk/downloads/statistics/mojstats/statistics-women-cjs-2010.pdf, accessed on 26 May 2012.

MoJ (2011) *Statistics on Race and the Criminal Justice System 2010. A Ministry of Justice Publication under Section 95 of the Criminal Justice Act 1991.* London: MoJ. Available at www.gov.uk/government/uploads/system/uploads/attachment_data/file/219967/stats-race-cjs-2010.pdf, accessed on 21 November 2013.

Montgomery, E. and Foldspang, A. (2008) 'Discrimination, mental problems and social adaptation in young refugees.' *European Journal of Public Health 199*, 2, 156–161.

Mooney, A., Statham, J., Monck, E. and Chambers, H. (2009) *Promoting the Health of Looked After Children: A Study to Inform Revision of the 2002 Guidance (Research Report No. DCSF-RR125, Institute of Education, University of London).* London: Department for Children, Schools and Families.

Mooney, G. and Neal, S. (2010) '"Welfare worries": Mapping the directions of welfare futures in the contemporary UK.' *Research, Policy and Planning 27*, 3, 141–150.

Morgan, A. and Swann, C. (2004) *Social Capital for Health: Issues of Definition, Measurement and Links to Health.* London: Health Development Agency.

Morgan, A. and Ziglio, E. (2007) 'Revitalising the evidence base for public health: An assets model.' *Global Health Promotion 14*, no. 2 suppl., 17–22.

Morris, J. (1997) 'Gone missing? Disabled children living away from their families.' *Disability & Society 12*, 2, 241–258.

Morris, M. D., Popper, S. T., Rodwell, T. C., Brodine, S. K. and Brouwer, K. C. (2009) 'Healthcare barriers of refugees post-resettlement.' *Journal of Community Health 34*, 529–538.

Morrissey, K., Daly, A., Clarke, G., O'Donoghue, C. and Ballas, D. (2012) 'A rural/urban comparison of psychiatric inpatient admissions in Ireland.' *Journal of Public Mental Health 11*, 209–213.

Mullen, P. E., Walton, V. A., Romans-Clarkson, S. E. and Herbison, G. P. (1988) 'Impact of sexual and physical abuse on women's mental health.' *The Lancet 331*, 8590, 841–845.

Murphy, E., Kapur, N., Webb, R., Purandare, N., *et al.* (2012) 'Risk factors for repetition and suicide following self-harm in older adults: Multicentre cohort study.' *British Journal of Psychiatry 200*, 399–404.

Murrison, A. (2010) *Fighting Fit: A Mental Health Plan for Servicemen and Veterans.* Available at www.gov.uk/government/uploads/system/uploads/attachment_data/file/27375/20101006_mental_health_Report.pdf, accessed on 12 January 2013.

National Centre for Social Research (NatCen) (2011) *Evaluation of the National Healthy Schools Programme: Final Report.* London: NatCen.

National Consumer Council and National Social Marketing Centre (2006) *It's our Health! Recognising the Potential of Effective Social Marketing.* London: National Consumer Council and National Social Marketing Centre. Available at www.thensmc.com/sites/default/files/ItsOurHealthJune2006.pdf, accessed on 18 July 2014.

National Crime Agency (n.d.) *Human Trafficking.* Available at www.nationalcrimeagency.gov.uk/crime-threats/human-trafficking. London: National Crime Agency , accessed on 12 April 2014.

National Institute on Drug Abuse (2010) *Cocaine: Abuse and Addiction.* Bethesda, Maryland: National Institute on Drug Abuse. Available at www.drugabuse.gov/publications/research-reports/cocaine-abuse-addiction, accessed on 18 June 2012.

National Working Group on Child Protection and Disability (2003) *It Doesn't Happen to Disabled Children: Child Protection and Disabled Children.* London: National Society for the Prevention of Cruelty to Children (NSPCC).

Naylor, C., Parsonage, M., McDaid, D., Knapp, M., Fossey, M. and Galea, A. (2012) *Long-term Conditions and Mental Health: The Cost of Co-morbidities.* London: The King's Fund.

National Collaborating Centre for Mental Health (NCCMH) (2004a) *Depression: Management of Depression in Primary and Secondary Care.* Leicester/London: The British Psychological Society and the Royal College of Psychiatrists.

NCCMH (2004b) *Eating Disorders: Core Interventions in the Treatment and Management of Anorexia Nervosa, Bulimia Nervosa and Related Eating Disorders. National Clinical Practice Guideline Number CG9.* Rushden: The British Psychological Society/Gaskell.

NCCMH (2004c) *Self-harm: The Short-term Physical and Psychological Management and Secondary Prevention of Self-harm in Primary and Secondary Care. National Clinical Practice Guideline Number 16.* Leicester and London: The British Psychological Society/Royal College of Psychiatrists.

NCCMH (2005) *Depression in Children and Young People: Identification and Management in Primary, Community and Secondary Care. National Clinical Practice Guideline Number 28.* Leicester and London: The British Psychological Society/Royal College of Psychiatrists.

NCCMH (2006) *Bipolar Disorder: The Management of Bipolar Disorder in Adults, Children and Adolescents, in Primary and Secondary Care. National Clinical Practice Guideline Number 38.* Leicester and London: The British Psychological Society/ Royal College of Psychiatrists.

NCCMH (2007) *Antenatal and Postnatal Mental Health.* Leicester and London: The British Psychological Society/Royal College of Psychiatrists.

NCCMH (2008) *Drug Misuse: Psychosocial Interventions. National Clinical Practice Guideline Number 51.* Leicester and London: The British Psychological Society/ Royal College of Psychiatrists.

NCCMH (2009) *Depression in Adults with a Chronic Physical Health Problem: Treatment and Management. National Clinical Practice Guideline Number 91.* Leicester and London: The British Psychological Society/Royal College of Psychiatrists.

NCCMH (2010a) *Antisocial Personality Disorder: Treatment, Management and Prevention. National Clinical Practice Guideline Number 77.* Leicester and London: The British Psychological Society/Royal College of Psychiatrists.

NCCMH (2010b) *Schizophrenia: The NICE Guideline on Core Interventions in the Treatment and Management of Schizophrenia in Adults in Primary and Secondary Care – Updated Edition. National Clinical Practice Guideline Number 82.* Leicester and London: The British Psychological Society/Royal College of Psychiatrists.

NCCMH (2011a) *Alcohol-use Disorders.* Leicester and London: The British Psychological Society/Royal College of Psychiatrists.

NCCMH (2011b) *Common Mental Health Disorders: Identification and Pathways to Care. NICE Clinical Guideline 123.* Leicester and London: The British Psychological Society/Royal College of Psychiatrists.

NCCMH (2011c) *Depression: The Treatment and Management of Depression in Adults –Updated Edition. National Clinical Practice Guideline Number 90.* Leicester and London: The British Psychological Society/Royal College of Psychiatrists.

NCCMH (2012a) *Improving the Experience of Care for People Using Adult NHS Mental Health Services. National Clinical Practice Guideline Number 136.* Leicester and London: The British Psychological Society/Royal College of Psychiatrists.

NCCMH (2012b) *Self-harm: Longer-Term Management. National Clinical Practice Guideline Number 133.* Leicester and London: The British Psychological Society/ Royal College of Psychiatrists.

National Confidential Inquiry into Suicide and Homicide by People with Mental Illness (NCI) (2013) *Annual Report: England, Northern Ireland, Scotland and Wales.* Manchester: University of Manchester.

New Economics Foundation (NEF) (2012) *Measuring Well-being: A Guide for Practitioners.* London: NEF.

North East Public Health Observatory (NEPHO) (2005) *The Health Needs of Prisoners.* Stockton-on-Tees: NEPHO.

NEPHO (2013) *Community Mental Health Profiles 2013.* Stockton-on-Tees: NEPHO. Available at www.nepho.org.uk/cmhp, accessed on 21 March 2014.

Nettle, D., Pepper, G. V., Jobling, R. and Schroeder, K. B. (2014) 'Being there: A brief visit to a neighbourhood induces the social attitudes of that neighbourhood.' *Peer J. doi: 10.7717/peerj.236.* Available at https://peerj.com/articles/236, accessed on 21 February 2014.

Newbronner, L., Chamberlains, R., Borthwick, R., Baxter, M. and Sanderson, D. (2013) *Sustaining and Spreading Self-Management Support – Lessons from Co-creating Health, Phase 2.* London: Health Foundation.

Newbury-Birch, D., Gilvarry, E., McArdle, P., Ramesh, V., *et al.* (2008) *Impact of Alcohol Consumption on Young People: A Review of Reviews.* Newcastle upon Tyne: Institute of Health and Society at Newcastle University.

NHS Choices (2012a) *Obesity.* NHS Choices. Available at www.nhs.uk/conditions/ Obesity/Pages/Introduction.aspx, accessed on 20 April 2014.

NHS Choices (2012b) *Veterans: Mental Health.* NHS Choices. Available at http:// webarchive.nationalarchives.gov.uk/+/www.nhs.uk/Livewell/Militarymedicine/ Pages/Veteransmentalhealth.aspx, accessed on 18 July 2013.

NHS Choices (n.d.) *Advice for Line Managers on Supporting Employees with Long-term Medical Conditions.* NHS Choices. Available at www.nhs.uk/Livewell/ workplacehealth/Documents/ChronicConds_LineManagers_Factsheet_A4.pdf, accessed on 18 July 2014.

NHS Confederation (2010) *Improving Mental Health Services for Veterans.* London: NHS Confederation.

NHS Confederation (2011) *From Illness to Wellness: Achieving Efficiencies and Improving Outcomes. Briefing 224.* London: NHS Confederation.

NHS Confederation (2012) *Community Health Champions: Creating New Relationships with Patients and Communities.* London/Wakefield: The NHS Confederation/ Altogether Better.

NHS Confederation (2013) *Good Practice in Joint Health and Wellbeing Strategies: A Self Evaluation Tool for Health and Wellbeing Boards.* NHS Confederation. Available at www.nhsconfed.org/HWB, accessed on 3 March 2014.

NHS England (2013) *News. New Staffing Guidance Published to Support Providers and Commissioners to Make the Right Decisions about Nursing, Midwifery and Care Staffing Capacity and Capability.* NHS England. Available at www.england.nhs. uk/2013/11/19/staff-guidance, accessed on 12 April 2014.

NHS Greater Glasgow and Clyde (2013) *Working with Asylum Seekers and Refugees/ Mental Health.* NHS Greater Glasgow and Clyde. Available at www.nhsggc.org.uk/ content/default.asp?page=s1094_1, accessed on 31 July 2013.

NHS Knowledge Services (2007) *Mental Health Risks of Obesity Drug. Behind the Headlines*. London: Department of Health. Available at www.nhs.uk/news/2007/November/Pages/Mentalhealthrisksofobesitydrug.aspx, accessed on 2 August 2013.

NHS Information Centre for Health and Social Care (NHSIC) (2009) *Adult Psychiatric Morbidity in England, 2007: Results of a Household Survey. A Survey Carried out for the NHS Information Centre for Health and Social Care by the National Centre for Social Research and Dept of Health Sciences, University of Leicester*. London: NHSIC/Social Care Statistics.

NHSIC (2010) *Survey of Carers in Households 2009/10*. London: NHSIC.

National Institute for Health and Clinical Excellence (now National Institute for Health and Care Excellence) (NICE) (2004a) *Guidance on Cancer Services. Improving Supportive and Palliative Care for Adults with Cancer*. London: NICE.

NICE (2004b) *Quick Reference Guide. Eating Disorders: Core Interventions in the Treatment and Management of Anorexia Nervosa, Bulimia Nervosa and Related Eating Disorders*. London: NICE.

NICE (2005) *Post-Traumatic Stress Disorder (PTSD): The Management of PTSD in Adults and Children in Primary and Secondary Care. Clinical Guideline 26*. London: NICE.

NICE (2006) *Health Equity Audit – Learning from Practice Briefing*. London: NICE.

NICE (2007) *Antenatal and Postnatal Mental Health (CG45)*. London: NICE.

NICE (2009a) *Depression in Adults: The Treatment and Management of Depression in Adults. Clinical Guideline 90*. London: NICE.

NICE (2009b) *Depression in Adults with a Chronic Physical Health Problem: Treatment and Management*. London: NICE.

NICE (2009c) *Managing Long-term Sickness and Incapacity for Work. NICE Public Health Guidance 19*. London: NICE.

NICE (2009d) *Promoting Mental Well-being at Work. NICE Public Health Guidance 22*. London: NICE.

NICE (2009e) *Social and Emotional Wellbeing in Secondary Education. NICE Public Health Guidance 20*. London: NICE.

NICE (2010) *Alcohol-use Disorders: Preventing Harmful Drinking. NICE Public Health Guidance 24*. London: NICE.

NICE (2011a) *Commissioning Stepped Care for People with Common Mental Health Disorders*. London: NICE.

NICE (2011b) *Common Mental Health Disorders: Identification and Pathways to Care. Clinical Guideline 123*. London: NICE.

NICE (2011c) *Depression in Adults. Quality Standard QS8*. London: NICE.

NICE (2012a) *Methods for the Development of NICE Public Health Guidance, Third Edition*. London: NICE.

NICE (2012b) *News: Tackle Mental Health Problems among those with Long-term Conditions, says Thinktank*. London: NICE.

NICE (2013a) *Social Anxiety Disorder: Recognition, Assessment and Treatment. Clinical Guideline 159*. London: NICE.

NICE (2013b) *Social Care of Older People with Multiple Long Term Conditions. Final Scope.* London: NICE.

NICE (2013c) *Tobacco: Harm-reduction Approaches to Smoking. NICE Public Health Guidance 45.* London: NICE.

NICE (2014) *Body Mass Index Threshold for Intervening to Prevent Ill Health among Black, Asian and Other Minority Ethnic Groups.* London: NICE.

NICE and Social Care Institute for Excellence (SCIE) (2010, modified April 2013) *Looked-after Children and Young People. NICE Public Health Guidance 28.* London: NICE.

Nicholls, A. (2006) *Assessing the Mental Health Needs of Older People.* London: Social Care Institute for Excellence.

Nicholls, J., Lawlor, E., Neitzert, E. and Goodspeed, T. (2012) *Guide to Social Return on Investment.* Haddington: The SROI Network.

Nicholson, L. A. (2008) 'Rural mental health.' *Advances in Psychiatric Treatment 14*, 302–311.

Nicholson, N. R. (2012) 'A review of social isolation: An important but underassessed condition in older people.' *Journal of Primary Prevention 33*, 2–3, 137–152.

National Institute for Mental Health in England (NIMHE) (2005) *Making it Possible: Improving Mental Health and Well-being in England.* London: NIMHE.

Nocon, A. (2004) *Background Evidence for the DRC's Formal Investigation into Health Inequalities Experienced by People with Learning Difficulties or Mental Health Problems.* London: Disability Rights Commission.

National Obesity Observatory (NOO) (2011) *Obesity and Ethnicity.* Oxford: National Obesity Observatory.

North East Climate Change Partnership (2008) *North East Climate Change Adaptation Study.* Available at www.climatenortheast.com/manageContent.aspx?object.id=10688, accessed on 28 October 2013.

National Society for the Prevention of Cruelty to Children (NSPCC) (2010) *ChildLine Casenotes: Children Talking to ChildLine about Loneliness.* London: NSPCC. Available at www.nspcc.org.uk/inform/publications/casenotes/clcasenotes_loneliness_wdf74260.pdf, accessed on 30 July 2013.

NSPCC (2011) *Casenotes: Looked After Children Talking to ChildLine.* London: NSPCC. Available at www.nspcc.org.uk/Inform/publications/casenotes/clcasenoteslookedafterchildren_wdf80622.pdf, accessed on 30 July 2013.

NSPCC (2013) *Female Genital Mutilation Helpline Launched.* London: NSPCC. Available at www.nspcc.org.uk/news-and-views/our-news/child-protection-news/female-genital-mutilation-helpline/fgm-helpline-launched_wda96863.html, accessed on 6 September 2013.

NSW Health (2001) *A Framework for Building Capacity to Improve Health.* Gladesville, NSW: NSW Health Department. Available at www.health.nsw.gov.au/pubs/2001/pdf/framework_improve.pdf, accessed on 18 July 2014.

Nulman, I., Rovet, J., Stewart, D. E., Wolpin, J., *et al.* (2002) 'Child development following exposure to tricyclic antidepressants of fluoxetine throughout fetal life: A prospective, controlled study.' *American Journal of Psychiatry 159*, 11, 1889–1895.

Nursing Theories (2012) *Stages of Change Model/Transtheoretical Model (TTM).* Current Nursing. Available at http://currentnursing.com/nursing_theory/transtheoretical_model.html, accessed on 6 October 2013.

Nutbeam, D. (2000) 'Health literacy as a public health goal: A challenge for contemporary health education and communication strategies into the 21st century.' *Health Promotion International 15*, 3, 259–267.

O'Hara, M. W. and Swain, A. M. (1996) 'Rates and risk of postpartum depression: A meta analysis.' *International Review of Psychiatry 8*, 1, 37–54.

O'Keefe, M., Hills, A., Doyle, M., McCreadie, C., *et al.* (2007) *UK Study of Abuse and Neglect of Older People. Prevalence Survey Report.* London: King's College London/National Centre for Social Research.

Oberleitner, L. M., Mandel, D. L. and Easton, C. J. (2013) 'Treatment of co-occurring alcohol dependence and perpetration of intimate partner violence: The role of anger expression.' *Journal of Substance Abuse Treatment 45*, 3, 313–318.

Obst, P. and Stafurik, J. (2010) 'Online we are all able bodied: Online psychological sense of community and social support found through membership of disability-specific websites promotes well-being for people living with a physical disability.' *Journal of Community & Applied Social Psychology 20*, 6, 525–531.

Olivier, D., Lubman, D. I. and Fraser, R. (2007) 'Tobacco smoking within psychiatric inpatient settings: Biopsychosocial perspective.' *Australian & New Zealand Journal of Psychiatry 41*, 572–580.

Office for National Statistics (ONS) (2008) *Social Trends. No. 38.* Basingstoke: Palgrave Macmillan.

ONS (2011a) *2010-based Period and Cohort Life Expectancy Tables.* London: ONS. Available at www.ons.gov.uk/ons/dcp171780_238828.pdf, accessed on 14 April 2013.

ONS (2011b) *National Population Projections, 2010-based Statistical Bulletin.* London: ONS. Available at www.ons.gov.uk/ons/dcp171778_235886.pdf, accessed on 14 April 2013.

ONS (2012a) *2011 Census: Usual Resident Population by Five-year Age Group and Sex, Local Authorities in the United Kingdom.* London: ONS. Available at www.ons.gov. uk/ons/rel/census/2011-census/population-and-household-estimates-for-the-united-kingdom/rft-table-3-census-2011.xls, accessed on 3 January 2013.

ONS (2012b) *Measuring National Well-being, Education and Skills.* London: ONS.

ONS (2013a) *Comparison of Mid-2010 Population Estimates by Ethnic Group Against the 2011 Census.* London: ONS. Available at www.ons.gov.uk/ons/rel/peeg/population-estimates-by-ethnic-group--experimental-/comparison-of-mid-2010-population-estimates-by-ethnic-group-against-the-2011-census/index.html, accessed on 17 April 2014.

ONS (2013b) *Focus on: Violent Crime and Sexual Offences, 2011/12*. London: ONS. Available at www.ons.gov.uk/ons/dcp171778_298904.pdf, accessed on 31 July 2013.

ONS (2013c) *Health Survey for England 2012*. London: HSCIS. Available at www.hscic. gov.uk/article/2021/Website-Search?productid=13887&q=HSE2012&sort=Relev ance&size=10&page=1&area=both#top, accessed on 18 July 2014.

ONS (2013d) *Leading Causes of Death. Part of Mortality Statistics: Deaths Registered in England and Wales (Series DR), 2012 Release*. London: ONS. Available at www. ons.gov.uk/ons/rel/vsob1/mortality-statistics--deaths-registered-in-england-and-wales--series-dr-/2012/info-causes-of-death.html, accessed on 10 April 2014.

ONS (2013e) *ONS Statistical Bulletin: Experimental Statistics. Personal Well-being across the UK, 2012/13*. London: ONS.

ONS (2013f) *ONS Statistical Bulletin: Suicides in the United Kingdom 2011*. London: ONS. Available at www.ons.gov.uk/ons/rel/subnational-health4/suicides-in-the-united-kingdom/2011/stb-suicide-bulletin.html, accessed on 24 March 2013.

Oswald, S. H., Heil, K. and Goldbeck, L. (2010) 'History of maltreatment and mental health problems in foster children: A review of the literature.' *Journal of Pediatric Psychology 35*, 5, 462–472.

Owen, C. and Stratham, J. (2009) *Disproportionality in Child Welfare*. London: Thomas Coram Research Unit/University of London/Department for Children, Schools and Families.

Oxford Dictionaries (n.d.) *Bully*. Oxford: Oxford University Press. Available at www. oxforddictionaries.com/definition/english/bully?q=bully, accessed on 26 July 2014.

Pachauri, R. K. and Reisinger, A. (eds) (2007) *IPCC Fourth Assessment Report: Climate Change 2007. Synthesis Report*. Geneva: Intergovernmental Panel on Climate Change (IPCC).

Parkinson, J. (2007) *Establishing a Core Set of National, Sustainable Mental Health Indicators for Adults in Scotland: Final Report*. Scotland: NHS Health Scotland.

Patton, G. C., Coffey, C., Carlin, J. B., Degenhardt, L., Lynskey, M. and Hall, W. (2002) 'Cannabis use and mental health in young people: Cohort study.' *British Medical Journal 325*, 1195–1198.

Paul, K. I. and Moser, K. (2009) 'Unemployment impairs mental health: Meta-analyses.' *Journal of Vocational Behaviour 74*, 3, 264–282.

Payne, S. (2000) *Poverty, Social Exclusion and Mental Health: Findings from the 1999 PSE Survey. Working Paper No. 15. Poverty and Social Exclusion Survey of Britain*. Bristol: Townsend Centre for International Poverty Research/University of Bristol.

Pearce, J. J., Williams, M. and Galvin, C. (2003) *The Choice and Opportunity Project: Young Women and Sexual Exploitation*. London: Joseph Rowntree Foundation.

Pearson, M. L., Mattke, S., Shaw, R., Ridgely, M. S. and Wiseman, S. H. (2007) *Patient Self-management Support Programs: An Evaluation*. Santa Monica, CA: Agency for Healthcare Research and Quality.

Penn, R. and Lambert, P. (2002) *Attitudes towards Ideal Family Size of Different Ethnic/ Nationality Groups in Great Britain, France and Germany. Population Trends 108*. London: ONS.

Phelan, M., Stradins, L. and Morrison, M. (2001) 'Physical health of people with severe mental illness.' *British Medical Journal 322*, 443–444.

Phillips, D. and Harrison, M. (2010) 'Constructing an integrated society: Historical lessons for tackling Black and Minority Ethnic housing segregation in Britain.' *Housing Studies 25*, 2, 221–235.

Phoenix, A. and Husain, F. (2007) *Parenting and Ethnicity*. York: Joseph Rowntree Foundation.

Pitt, M. (2008) *Learning Lessons from the 2007 Floods – Full Report*. London: The Cabinet Office. Available at http://webarchive.nationalarchives.gov.uk/20080906001345/www.cabinetoffice.gov.uk/~/media/assets/www.cabinetoffice.gov.uk/flooding_review/pitt_review_full%20pdf.ashx, accessed on 28 April 2013.

Plan (n.d.) *Early and Forced Marriage – Facts, Figures and What You Can Do*. Woking, Surrey: Plan. Available at www.plan-uk.org/early-and-forced-marriage, accessed on 13 March 2014.

Polivy, J. (1996) 'Psychological consequences of food restriction.' *Journal of the American Dietetic Association 96*, 6, 589–592.

Portes, A. (1998) 'Social capital: Its origins and applications in modern sociology.' *Annual Review of Sociology 24*, 1–24.

Prescott-Clarke, P. and Primatesta, P. (1998) *Health Survey for England '96*. London: TSO.

Prison Reform Trust (2011) *Bromley Briefings Prison Factfile*. London: Prison Reform Trust. Available at www.prisonreformtrust.org.uk/Portals/0/Documents/Bromley%20Briefing%20December%202011.pdf, accessed on 17 July 2014.

Prison Reform Trust (2012) *Bromley Briefings Prison Factfile June 2012*. London: Prison Reform Trust. Available at www.thebromleytrust.org.uk/Indexhibit/files/BromleyBriefingsJune2012.pdf, accessed on 17 July 2014

Prochaska, J. O. and DiClemente, C. C. (1984) *The Transtheoretical Approach: Towards a Systematic Eclectic Framework*. Homewood, IL: USA Dow Jones Irwin.

Prochaska, J. O., Velicer, W. F., Rossi, J. S., Goldstein, M. G., *et al*. (1994) 'Stages of change and decisional balance for 12 problem behaviors.' *Health Psychology 13*, 39–46.

Public Health Agency (2010) *Health Promoting Hospitals and Health Services Network in Northern Ireland – Update Report 2008–09*. Belfast: Public Health Agency. Available at www.publichealth.hscni.net/sites/default/files/Health%20Promoting%20Hospitals% 20Report%202008-2009.pdf, accessed on 30 September 2013.

Public Health Policy and Strategy Unit (2013) *Healthy Lives, Healthy People Public Health Workforce Strategy 2013*. London: DH, PHE (Public Health England) and LGA (Local Government Association). Available at www.gov.uk/government/publications/healthy-lives-healthy-people-a-public-workforce-strategy, accessed on 30 September 2013.

Putnam, R. (1993) *Making Democracy Work: Civic Traditions in Modern Italy*. Princeton, NJ: Princeton University Press.

Putting People First (n.d.) *Personalisation Communications Toolkit*. London: Think Local Act Personal. Available at www.thinklocalactpersonal.org.uk/_library/Resources/Personalisation/Localmilestones/Putting_People_First_Communications_Toolkit.pdf, accessed on 8 June 2013.

Quarmby, K. (2011) *Scapegoat: Why we are Failing Disabled People*. London: Portobello Books Limited.

Qureshi, S. U., Pyne, J. M., Magruder, K. M., Schulz, P. E. and Kunik, M. E. (2009) 'The link between post-traumatic stress disorder and physical comorbidities: A systematic review.' *Psychiatric Quarterly 80*, 2, 87–97.

Radford, J., Harne, L. and Trotter, J. (2006) 'Disabled women and domestic violence as violent crime.' *Practice: Social Work in Action 18*, 4, 233–246.

Raghavan, R. and Pawson, N. (2009) *Meeting the Leisure Needs of Young People with a Learning Disability from South Asian Communities*. London: Mencap.

Ramrakha, S., Caspi, A., Dickson, N., Moffitt, T. E. and Paul, C. (2000) 'Psychiatric disorders and risky sexual behaviour in young adulthood: Cross sectional study in birth cohort.' *BMJ 321*, 263.

Rand, M. L. R. and Harrel, E. (2007) *Crime Against People with Disabilities*. Lincoln: US Department of Justice at DigitalCommons@University of Nebraska. Available at http://digitalcommons.unl.edu/cgi/viewcontent.cgi?article=1024&context=usjusticematls, accessed on 6 December 2013.

Ratner, P. A. (1993) 'The incidence of wife abuse and mental health status in abused wives in Edmonton, Alberta.' *Canadian Journal of Public Health 84*, 4, 246–249.

Royal College of Midwives (RCM), Royal College of Nursing (RCN), Royal College of Obstetricians and Gynaecologists (RCOG), Equality Now, Community Practitioners and Health Visitors Association (CPHVA) and UNITE (2013) *Tackling FGM in the UK: Intercollegiate Recommendations for Identifying, Recording, and Reporting*. London: RCM.

Royal College of Nursing (RCN) (2010) *Health and Nursing Care in the Criminal Justice Service*. London: RCN.

RCN (2013) *RCN Fact Sheet: Clinical Commissioning Groups*. London: RCN. Available at www.rcn.org.uk/__data/assets/pdf_file/0019/502714/7.13_RCN_Fact_sheet_on_Clinical_commissioning_groups_April_2013.pdf, accessed on 18 April 2014.

Royal College of Psychiatrists (RCPsych) (2009) *Cannabis and Mental Health*. London: RCPsych. Available at www.rcpsych.ac.uk/mentalhealthinfoforall/problems/alcoholanddrugs/cannabisandmentalhealth.aspx, accessed on 18 June 2012.

RCPsych (2010) *Self-harm, Suicide and Risk: Helping People Who Self-Harm. Final Report of a Working Group (College Report CR158)*. London: RCPsych.

Rees, G., Goswami, H., Pople, L., Bradshaw, J., Keung, A. and Main, G. (2012) *Good Childhood Report*. Leeds: The Children's Society.

Regional Youth Work Unit and Save the Children (2003) *Review of Youth Work with Black and Minority Ethnic Young People in Newcastle upon Tyne*. Newcastle: Newcastle City Council's Play and Youth Service.

Remafedi, G., French, S., Story, M., Resnick, M. D. and Blum, R. (1998) 'The relationship between suicide risk and sexual orientation: Results of a population-based study.' *American Journal of Public Health 88*, 1, 57–60.

Repper, J. and Breeze, J. (2006) 'User and carer involvement in the training and education of health professionals: A review of the literature.' *International Journal of Nursing Studies 44*, 511–519.

Repper, R., Simpson, A. and Grimshaw, G. (2011) *Good Practice Guide for Involving Carers, Family Members and Close Friends of Service Users in Research*. London: Mental Health Research Network/National Institute for Health Research.

Rethink (2004) *Only the Best*. London: Rethink.

Richard, M. and Huppert, F. A. (2011) 'Do positive children become positive adults? Evidence from a longitudinal birth cohort study.' *Journal of Positive Psychology 6*, 1, 75–87.

Rissell, C. (1994) 'Empowerment: The holy grail of health promotion?' *Health Promotion International 9*, 1, 39–45.

Robertson, E., Jones, I. and Haque, S. (2004) 'Antenatal risk factors for postpartum depression: A synthesis of recent literature.' *General Hospital Psychiatry 26*, 289–295.

Robotham, D., Morgan, K. and James, K. (2011) *Learning for Life. Adult Learning, Mental Health and Wellbeing*. London: Mental Health Foundation. Available at www.mentalhealth.org.uk/content/assets/PDF/publications/learning-for-life.pdf, accessed on 27 August 2013.

Rodger, E. and Chappel, D. (2008) *NEPHO Occasional Paper No. 29. Migrant Health in North East England*. Thornaby-on-Tees: North East Public Health Observatory.

Romans, S. E., Poore, M. R. and Martin, J. L. (2000) 'The perpetrators of domestic violence.' *Medical Journal of Australia 173*, 9, 484–488.

Roulstone, A., Thomas, P. and Balderston, S. (2011) 'Between hate and vulnerability: Unpacking the British criminal justice system's construction of disablist hate crime.' *Disability & Society 26*, 3, 351–364.

Russell, D. (2009) 'Living arrangements, social integration, and loneliness in later life: The case of physical disability.' *Journal of Health and Social Behavior 50*, 4, 460–475.

Russell, L., Thompson, R. and Simmons, R. (2014) *Helping Unemployed Young People to Find Private Sector Work*. York: Joseph Rowntree Foundation.

Rutherford, K., McIntyre, J., Daley, A. and Ross, L. E. (2012) 'Development of expertise in mental health service provision for lesbian, gay, bisexual and transgender communities.' *Medical Education 46*, 9, 903–913.

Ryan, C., Russell, S. T., Huebner, D., Diaz, R. and Sanchez, J. (2010) 'Family acceptance in adolescence and the health of LGBT young adults.' *Journal of Child and Adolescent Psychiatric Nursing 23*, 4, 205–213.

Ryan, D. and Kostaras, X. (2005) 'Psychiatric disorders in the post partum period.' *BC Medical Journal 47*, 2, 100–103.

Salway, S., Platt, L., Chowbey, P., Harriss, K. and Bayliss, E. (2007) *Long-term Ill Health, Poverty and Ethnicity*. York: Joseph Rowntree Foundation.

Scottish Association for Mental Health (SAMH) (2012) *Know Where to Go. SAMH Research Report: Remote and Rural Mental Health. Glasgow:* SAMH. Available at www.samh.org.uk/media/287333/know_where_to_go_-_remote__rural_report_final.pdf, accessed on 31 July 2013.

Sardar, Z. (2008) 'First person.' *The Guardian,* 13 September 2008. Available at www.theguardian.com/lifeandstyle/2008/sep/13/family1, accessed on 17 April 2014.

Standing Conference for Community Development (SCCD) (2001) *The Strategic Framework for Community Development.* Falkland, Fife: International Association for Community Development. Available at www.iacdglobal.org/files/sframepdf.pdf, accessed on 7 August 2013.

Scottish Community Development Centre for Learning Connections (SCDCLC) (2007) *Building Community Capacity: Resources for Community Learning and Development Practice. An Introductory Guide.* Edinburgh: The Scottish Government.

Schmuecker, K. (2014) *Future of the UK Labour Market.* York: Joseph Rowntree Foundation.

Schuller, N. (2005) 'Disabled people, crime and social isolation.' *Community Safety Journal 4,* 3, 4–13.

Social Care Institute of Excellence (SCIE) (2005) *The Health and Wellbeing of Young Carers.* London: SCIE.

SCIE (2011) *Preventing Loneliness and Social Isolation: Interventions and Outcomes.* London: SCIE.

Sainsbury Centre for Mental Health (SCMH) (2007) *Mental Health at Work: Developing the Business Case.* London: SCMH.

Scott, K. M., Bruffaaerts, R., Simon, G. E., Alonson, J., et al. (2008) 'Obesity and mental disorders in the general population: Results from the world mental health surveys.' *International Journal of Obesity 32,* 192–200.

Scottish Community Development Centre (2011) *Community Development and Co-production: Issues for Policy and Practice.* Glasgow: Scottish Community Development Centre.

Scottish Government, The (2004) *Children and Young People's Mental Health: A Framework for Promotion, Prevention and Care.* Edinburgh: Scottish Executive. Available at www.scotland.gov.uk/Publications/2004/12/20383/48310, accessed on 19 September 2014.

Scottish Government, The (2007) *Towards a Mentally Flourishing Scotland: The Future of Mental Health Improvement in Scotland 2008–11.* Edinburgh: The Scottish Government. Available at www.scotland.gov.uk/Publications/2007/10/26112853/7, accessed on 24 July 2014.

Scottish Government, The (2008) *Living and Dying Well: A National Action Plan for Palliative and End of Life Care for Adults in Scotland.* Edinburgh: The Scottish Government. Available at www.scotland.gov.uk/Resource/Doc/239823/0066155.pdf, accessed on 17 July 2013.

Scottish Government, The (2009) *Improving the Health & Wellbeing of People with Long Term Conditions in Scotland: A National Action Plan. CEL 23.* Edinburgh: The Scottish Government. Available at www.sehd.scot.nhs.uk/mels/CEL2009_23.pdf, accessed on 5 December 2013.

Scottish Government, The (2012a) *Child and Adolescent Mental Health.* Edinburgh: The Scottish Government. Available at www.scotland.gov.uk/ Publications/2012/08/9714/6, accessed on 23 February 2014.

Scottish Government, The (2012b) *National Outcomes.* Edinburgh: The Scottish Government. Available at www.scotland.gov.uk/About/Performance/ scotPerforms/outcomes, accessed on 26 February 2012.

Scottish Government, The (2012c) *Community Care Outcomes Framework.* Edinburgh: The Scottish Government.

Scottish Government, The (2012d) *Mental Health Strategy for Scotland 2012–2015.* Edinburgh: The Scottish Government.

Scottish Government, The (2013) *Scottish Health Survey 2012.* Edinburgh: The Scottish Government.

Scottish Government, The and Convention of Scottish Local Authorities (COSLA) (2012) *Single Outcome Agreements: Guidance to Community Planning Partnerships.* Edinburgh: The Scottish Government. Available at www.scotland.gov.uk/Topics/ Government/local-government/CP/SOA2012/SOA2012, accessed on 14 April 2014.

Scottish Parliamentary Corporate Body (2013) *Public Bodies (Joint Working) (Scotland) Bill – Explanatory Notes (and other accompanying documents).* Edinburgh: Scottish Parliamentary Corporate Body.

Seddon, J. (2012) 'Foreword.' In C. Pell (ed.) *Delivering Public Services that Work. Volume 2 The Vanguard Method in the Public Sector: Case Studies.* Devon: Triarchy Press.

Seebohm, P. (2008) *Evening the Odds: Employment Support, Mental Health and Black and Minority Ethnic Communities. Briefing Paper 35.* London: SCMH.

Seebohm, P., Henderson, P., Munn-Giddings, C., Thomas, P. and Yasmeen, S. (2005) *Together We Will Change – Community Development, Mental Health and Diversity.* Bradford: Sharing Voices.

Seedhouse, D. (1988) *Ethics: The Heart of Health Care, Second Edition.* Chichester: John Wiley and Sons.

Seel, D. (2008) *Introduction to Appreciative Inquiry.* New Paradigm Consulting. Available at www.new-paradigm.co.uk/introduction_to_ai.htm, accessed on 21 July 2013.

Shahab, L. and West, R. (2009) 'Do ex-smokers report feeling happier following cessation? Evidence from a cross-sectional survey.' *Nicotine and Tobacco Research 11*, 5, 553–557.

Sharp, C., McConville, S. and Tompkins, C. (2011) *Evaluation of Keep Well in Prisons.* Glasgow: NHS Health Scotland.

Shear, M. K., Simon, N., Wall, M., Zisook, S., *et al.* (2011) 'Complicated grief and related bereavement issues for DSM-5.' *Depression and Anxiety 28*, 2, 103–117.

Shewell, D. and Penn, D. (2005) *Equality and Diversity in the North East Region of England: A Baseline Study*. Newcastle upon Tyne: North East Regional Information Partnership (NERIP).

Shortus, T., Kemp, L., McKenzie, S. and Harris, M. (2013) 'Managing patient involvement: Provider perspectives on diabetes decision-making.' *Health Expectations 16*, 2, 189–198.

Shribman, S. and Billingham, K. (2009) *Healthy Child Programme: Pregnancy and the First 5 Years of Life*. London: DH.

Shub, D. and Kunik, M. E. (2009) 'Psychiatric comorbidity in persons with dementia: assessment and treatment strategies.' *Psychiatric Times 26*. Available at www.psychiatrictimes.com/articles/comorbidity-psychiatric-comorbidity-persons-dementia, accessed on 17 July 2014.

Sigerson, D. and Gruer, L. (2011) *Asset-based Approaches to Health Improvement*. Glasgow: NHS Health Scotland.

Sigona, N. and Hughes, V. (2012) *No Way Out, No Way In: Irregular Migrant Children and Families in the UK*. Oxford: The Economic and Social Research Council (ESRC) Centre on Migration, Policy and Society/University of Oxford.

Simon, J. and Rosolova, H. (2002) 'Family history – and independent risk factors for coronary heart disease, it is time to be practical.' *European Heart Journal 23*, 1637–1638.

Simpson, E. L. and House, A. O. (2003) 'User and carer involvement in mental health services: From rhetoric to science.' *British Journal of Psychiatry 183*, 89–91.

Singleton, N. and Lewis, G. (eds) (2003) *Better or Worse: A Longitudinal Study of the Mental Health of Adults Living in Private Households in Great Britain*. London: TSO.

Singleton, N., Maung, N. A., Cowie, A., Sparks, J., Bumpstead, R. and Meltzer, H. (2002) *Mental Health of Carers*. London: ONS.

Sissons, P. and Jones, K. (2014) *How Can Local Skills Strategies Help Low Earners?* York: Joseph Rowntree Foundation.

Skeg, K., Nada-Raja, S., Dickson, N., Paul, C. and Williams, S. (2003) 'Sexual orientation and self-harm in men and women.' *American Journal of Psychiatry 160*, 3, 541–546.

Skocpol, T. (1996) 'Unravelling from above.' *The American Prospect 7*, 25, 20–25.

Sleijpen, M., ter Heide, F. J. J. and Kleber, R. J. (2013) 'Bouncing forward of young refugees: A perspective on resilience research direction.' *European Journal of Psychotraumatology 4*. Available at www.ncbi.nlm.nih.gov/pmc/articles/PMC3644055, accessed on 9 March 2014.

Smith, N. and Middleton, S. (2007) *A Review of Poverty Dynamics Research in the UK*. York: Joseph Rowntree Foundation.

Smith, S. M., Soubhi, J., Fortin, M., Hudon, C. and O'Dowd, T. (2012) 'Interventions for improving outcomes in patients with multimorbidity in primary care and community settings.' *Cochrane Database of Systematic Reviews 4*. Article Number: CD006560.

Smithies, J. and Webster, G. (1998) *Community Involvement in Health: From Passive Recipients to Active Participants*. Aldershot: Ashgate.

Social Exclusion Unit (2002) *Reducing Re-offending by Ex-Prisoners.* London: Social Exclusion Unit.

Social Exclusion Unit (2004) *Mental Health and Social Exclusion.* London: Office of the Deputy Prime Minister (ODPM).

Sorkin, D., Rook, J. L. and Lu, J. L. (2002) 'Loneliness, lack of emotional support, lack of companionship, and the likelihood of having a heart condition in an elderly sample.' *Annals of Behavioral Medicine 24,* 4, 290–298.

South, J., White, J. and Woodall, J. (2010) *Altogether Better. Community Health Champions and Empowerment: Thematic Evaluation Summary.* Leeds: Centre for Health Promotion Research/Leeds Metropolitan University.

SSIA (Social Services Improvement Agency) (2011) *What Works in Promoting Good Outcomes for Children in Need Who Experience Domestic Violence?* Cardiff: SSIA. Available at www.ssiacymru.org.uk/resource/g_a_Promoting_Good_Outcomes_for_Children_who_experience_Domestic_Violence.pdf, accessed 20 July 2014.

St Leger, L. (2001) 'Schools, health literacy and public health: Possibilities and challenges.' *Health Promotion International 16,* 2, 197–205.

St Mungo's (2008) *Homelessness: It Makes You Sick.* London: St Mungo's.

Stalker, K. and Moscardini, L. (2012) *A Critical Review and Analysis of Current Research and Policy Relating to Disabled Children and Young People in Scotland. A Report to Scotland's Commissioner for Children and Young People.* Glasgow: University of Strathclyde.

Stark, E., Flitcraft, A., Zuckerman, B., Grey, A., Robinson, J. and Frazier, W. (1981) *Wife Abuse in the Medical Setting: An Introduction for Health Personnel.* Washington DC: Department of Health and Human Services, Office of Child Abuse and Neglect.

Steele, A. and Ahmed, N. (2007) *Homelessness among Black Communities in the London Borough of Islington.* London: London Borough of Islington.

Stephens, L., Ryan-Collins, J. and Boyle, D. (2008) *Co-production: A Manifesto for Growing the Core Economy.* London: NEF.

Stern, N. H. (2007) *The Economics of Climate Change: The Stern Review.* Cambridge, UK: Cambridge University Press.

Stevens, A., Raftery, J., Mant, J. and Simpson, S. (2004) *Health Care Needs Assessment: The Epidemiologically Based Needs Assessment Reviews.* Oxford/San Francisco, CA: Radcliffe Publishing.

Stewart-Brown, S. (2002) 'Interpersonal relationships and the origins of mental health.' *Journal of Public Mental Health 4,* 1, 24–29.

Strand, S. (1999) 'Ethnic group, sex and economic disadvantage: Associations with pupils' educational progress from baseline to the end of Key Stage 1.' *British Educational Research Journal 25,* 2, 179–202.

Strand, S. (2008) *Minority Ethnic Pupils in the Longitudinal Study of Young People in England. Report DCSF-RR029.* London: Department for Children, Schools and Families.

Stuart, H. (2006) 'Mental illness and employment discrimination.' *Current Opinion in Psychiatry 19,* 5, 522.

Stuckler, D. and Basu, S. (2013) *The Body Economic: Why Austerity Kills*. New York, NY: Basic Books.

Stuckler, D., King, L. and McKee, M. (2009) 'Mass privatisation and the post-communist mortality crisis: A cross-national analysis.' *Lancet 373*, 399–407.

Substance Use and Mental Illness Treatment Team (2009) *Heroin and Mental Health*. Melbourne: NorthWestern Mental Health.

Sugiyama, T., Leslie, E., Giles-Corti, B. and Owen, N. (2008) 'Associations of neighbourhood greenness with physical and mental health: Do walking, social coherence and local social interaction explain the relationships?' *Journal of Epidemiology & Community Health*. doi: 10.1136/jech.2007.064287. Available at http://jech.bmj.com/content/62/5/e9.full.pdf+html?sid=371e09f3-403e-4c15-a715-376ea6c44ef0, accessed on 17 April 2014.

Suglia, S. F., Duarte, C. S. and Sandel, M. T. (2011) 'Housing quality, housing instability and maternal mental health.' *Journal of Urban Health 8*, 6, 1105–1116.

Swanton, K. (2008) *Healthy Weight, Healthy Lives: A Toolkit for Developing Local Strategies*. London: DH Publications.

Tackey, N. D., Barnes, H. and Khambhaita, P. (2011) *Poverty, Ethnicity and Education*. York: Joseph Rowntree Foundation.

Tackey, N. D., Casebourne, J., Aston, J., Ritchie, H., *et al.* (2006) *Barriers to Employment for Pakistanis and Bangladeshis in Britain. Research Report No 360*. Leeds: Department for Work and Pensions.

Tait, L. and Lester, H. (2005) 'Encouraging user involvement in mental health services.' *Advances in Psychiatric Treatment 11*, 168–175.

Tameside and Glossop Clinical Commissioning Group (2012) *5 Ways to Wellbeing*. Manchester: Tameside and Glossop CCG. Available at www.tamesideandglossopccg.org/campaigns/5-ways-to-wellbeing?site_locale=en, accessed on 13 December 2013.

Taylor, C. (2012) *Improving Attendance at School*. London: Department for Education.

Taylor, K. (2009) 'Asylum seekers, refugees and the politics of access to healthcare: A UK perspective.' *British Journal of General Practice 59*, 567, 765–772.

Taylor, K. (2012) *Primary Care: Working Differently. Telecare and Telehealth: A Game Changer for Health and Social Care*. London: Deloitte Centre for Health Solutions.

Taylor, K., Naylor, H., George, R. and Hammett, S. (2012) *Healthcare for the Homeless*. London: Deloitte Centre for Health Solutions.

Taylor, L., Taske, N., Swann, C. and Seymour, L. (2007) *Public Health Interventions to Promote Positive Mental Health and Prevent Mental Health Disorders among Adults. Evidence Briefing*. London: NICE.

Taylor, M. (2008) *Transforming Disadvantaged Places: Effective Strategies for Places and People*. York: Joseph Rowntree Foundation.

Tehrani, N. (2005) *Bullying at Work: Beyond Policies to a Culture of Respect*. London: Chartered Institute of Personnel and Development.

Thaler, R. H. and Sunstein, C. R. (2008, reprinted 2009) *Nudge: Improving Decisions about Health, Wealth and Happiness*. London: Penguin Books.

Thomas, C. (2013) *Adoption for Looked after Children: Messages from Research*. London: British Association for Adoption and Fostering.

Thomas, P., Seebohm, P., Henderson, P. K., Munn-Giddings, C. and Yasmeen, S. (2006) 'Tackling race inequalities: Community development, mental health and diversity.' *Journal of Public Mental Health* 5, 2, 13–19.

Tinker, A., Kellaher, L., Ginn, J. and Ribe, E. (2013) *Assisted Living Platform – The Long Term Care Revolution*. London: Institute of Gerontology, Department of Social Science, Health and Medicine, King's College London.

Together for Short Lives (2012) *A Guide to End of Life Care: Care of Children and Young People Before Death, at the Time of Death and After Death*. Bristol: Together for Short Lives. Available at www.togetherforshortlives.org.uk/assets/0000/1855/TfSL_A_Guide_to_End_of_Life_Care_5_FINAL_VERSION.pdf, accessed on 17 April 2014.

Townend, M. (2007) *Assertiveness Training*. Cognitive Behavioural Therapy. Available at www.cognitivebehaviourtherapy.co.uk/Assertiveness/page_01.htm, accessed on 20 August 2013.

Townsend, P. and Davidson, N. (eds) (1982) *Inequalities in Health: The Black Report*. Harmondsworth: Penguin Books Ltd.

Tribe, R. (2002) 'Mental health of refugees and asylum-seekers.' *Advances in Psychiatric Treatment* 8, 240–247.

Trivedi, D., Bunn, F., Graham, M. and Wentz, R. (2007) *Update on Review of Reviews on Teenage Pregnancy and Parenthood*. Hatfield: Centre for Research in Primary and Community Care, University of Hertfordshire on behalf of the National Institute for Health and Clinical Excellence.

University College London (UCL) Institute of Health Equity (2012) *The Impact of the Economic Downturn on Health Inequalities in London*. London: UCL. Available at www.instituteofhealthequity.org, accessed on 8 December 2013.

University of California, Los Angeles (UCLA) Center for Health Policy Research (n.d.) *Asset Mapping*. Los Angeles: UCLA Center for Health Policy Research. Available at http://healthpolicy.ucla.edu/programs/health-data/trainings/Documents/tw_cba20.pdf, accessed on 21 July 2013.

UK Collaborative Group for HIV and STI Surveillance, The (2006) *A Complex Picture: HIC and Other Sexually Transmitted Diseases in the United Kingdom*. London: Health Protection Agency.

United Nations Children's Fund (UNICEF) (2006) *Behind Closed Doors: The Impact of Domestic Violence on Children*. New York: UNICEF. Available at www.unicef.org/protection/files/BehindClosedDoors.pdf, accessed on 17 July 2014.

UNICEF (2013) *Female Genital Cutting/Circumcision: A Statistical Overview and Exploration of the Dynamics of Change*. New York, NY: UNICEF.

UNISON (2013) *Welfare Reform Changes Affecting Disabled People*. London: UNISON. Available at www.unison.org.uk/upload/sharepoint/On%20line%20Catalogue/21709.pdf, accessed on 6 December 2013.

United Nations General Security Council (1992) *An Agenda for Peace, Preventive Diplomacy, Peacemaking and Peace-keeping*. New York, NY: United Nations. Available at www.unrol.org/files/A_47_277.pdf, accessed on 20 July 2014.

United Nations High Commissioner for Refugees (2012) *A Year of Crisis: Global Trends 2011.* Geneva: UNHCR. Available at www.unhcr.org/4fd6f87f9.html, accessed on 23 January 2014.

United Nations Population Fund (2012) *Marrying Too Young.* New York, NY: United Nations Population Fund. Available at www.unfpa.org/webdav/site/global/shared/documents/publications/2012/MarryingTooYoung.pdf, accessed on 13 March 2014.

Utz-Billing, I. and Kentenich, H. (2008) 'Female genital mutilation: An injury, physical and mental harm.' *Journal of Psychosomatic Obstetrics & Gynecology 29*, 4, 225–229.

van den Berg, A. E., Maas, J., Verheij, R. A. and Groenewegen, P. P. (2010) 'Green space as a buffer between stressful life events and health.' *Social Science & Medicine 70*, 80, 1203–1210.

Vanstraelen, M., Holt, G. and Bouras, N. (1997) 'Adults with Learning Disabilities and Psychiatric Problems.' In W. Fraser and M. Kerr (eds) *Seminars in the Psychiatry of Learning Disabilities, Second Edition.* London: Royal Society of Psychiatrists.

Vass, J. (2013) *Agenda for Later Life: Improving Later Life in Tough Times.* London: Age UK.

Vloeberghs, E., van der Kwaak, A., Knipscheer, J. and van den Muijsenbergh, M. (2012) 'Coping and chronic psychosocial consequences of female genital mutilation in the Netherlands.' *Ethnicity & Health 17*, 6, 677–695.

Von Stumm, S., Deary, I. J., Kivimäki, M., Jokela, M., Clark, H. and Batty, G. D. (2011) 'Childhood behavior problems and health at mid-life: 35-year follow-up of a Scottish birth cohort.' *Journal of Child Psychology and Psychiatry 53*, 9, 992–1001.

Waddell, G. and Burton, A. K. (2006) *Is Work Good for Your Health and Well-being?* Norwich: TSO.

Wadhwa, P. D., Sandman, C. A., Porto, M., Dunkel-Schetter, C. and Garite, T. J. (1993) 'The association between prenatal stress and infant birthweight and gestational age at birth: A prospective investigation.' *American Journal of Obstetrics and Gynaecology 169*, 858–865.

Wahl, O. E., Wood, A. and Richards, R. (2002) 'Newspaper coverage of mental illness: Is it changing?' *Psychiatric Rehabilitation Skills 6*, 9–31.

Walby, S. and Allen, J. (2004) *Domestic Violence, Sexual Assault and Stalking: Findings from the British Crime Survey. Home Office Research Study No. 276.* London: Home Office.

Wallace, L. M., Turner, A., Kosmala-Anderson, J., Sharma, S., *et al.* (2012) *Co-creating Health: Evaluation of First Phase.* London: The Health Foundation.

Wanless, D. (2002) *Securing our Future Health: Taking a Long-term View. Final Report.* London: HM Treasury.

Warburton Brown, C. (2011) *Exploring BME Maternal Poverty. Oxfam GB Research Report.* Cowley: Oxfam GB.

Weaver, T., Hickman, M., Rutter, D., Ward, J., Stimson, G. and Renton, A. (2001) 'The prevalence and management of co-morbid substance misuse and mental illness: Results of a screening survey in substance misuse and mental health treatment populations.' *Drug and Alcohol Review 20*, 4, 407–416.

Webb, R., Abel, K., Pickles, A. and Appleby, L. (2005) 'Mortality in offspring of parents with psychotic disorders: A critical review and meta-analysis.' *American Journal of Psychiatry 162*, 6, 1045–1056.

Weich, S. and Lewis, G. (1998) 'Poverty, unemployment and common mental disorders: Population based cohort study.' *British Medical Journal 317*, 115–119.

Wellock, V. K. (2010) 'Domestic abuse: Black and minority-ethnic women's perspectives.' *Midwifery 26*, 2, 181–188.

Welsh Assembly Government (2009) *Talk to Me: The National Action Plan to Reduce Suicide and Self Harm in Wales 2009–2014.* Cardiff: Welsh Assembly Government.

Welsh Government (2012) *Together for Mental Health: A Strategy for Mental Health and Wellbeing in Wales.* Cardiff: Welsh Government.

Welsh Government (2013a) *Welsh Health Survey 2012.* Cardiff: Welsh Government.

Welsh Government (2013b) *General Medical Contract: Quality Outcomes Framework.* Cardiff: Welsh Government. Available at http://wales.gov.uk/statistics-and-research/general-medical-services-contract/?lang=en, accessed on 23 February 2014.

Welsh Government (2014) *NHS Outcomes Framework.* Cardiff: Welsh Government. Available at http://wales.gov.uk/about/cabinet/cabinetstatements/2013/8247136/?lang=en, accessed on 23 February 2014.

Welsh Government (n.d.) *Psychiatric Census.* Cardiff: Welsh Government. Available at https://statswales.wales.gov.uk/Catalogue/Health-and-Social-Care/Mental-Health/Psychiatric-Census, accessed on 23 February 2014.

West, R. and Jarvis, M. (2005) 'Tobacco smoking and mental disorder.' *Italian Journal of Psychiatry & Behavioural Science 15*, 10–17.

Women's Health and Equality Consortium (WHEC) (2013) *Better Health for Women: How to Incorporate Women's Health Needs into Joint Strategic Needs Assessments and Joint Health and Wellbeing Strategies.* London: WHEC. Available at www.whec.org.uk, accessed on 29 May 2013.

Whitelaw, S., Swift, J., Goodwin, G. and Clark, D. (2008) *Physical Activity and Mental Health: The Role of Physical Activity in Promoting Mental Wellbeing and Preventing Mental Health Problems. An Evidence Briefing.* Edinburgh: NHS Health Scotland.

Whitrow, M. J., Harding, S. and Maynard, M. J. (2010) 'The influence of parental smoking and family type on saliva cotinine in UK ethnic minority children: A cross sectional study.' *BMC Public Health 10*, 262.

World Health Organization (WHO) (1948) *Constitution of the World Health Organization.* Geneva: WHO.

WHO (1986) *The Ottawa Charter for Health Promotion.* Geneva: WHO.

WHO (1989) *Health Principles of Housing.* Geneva: WHO.

WHO (2009a) *7th Global Conference on Health Promotion: Track Themes. Track 2: Health Literacy and Health Behaviour.* Geneva: WHO. Available at www.who.int/healthpromotion/conferences/7gchp/track2/en, accessed on 26 August 2013.

WHO (2009b) *Milestones in Health Promotion. Statements from Global Conferences.* Geneva: WHO.

WHO (2010) *Global Strategy to Stop Health-care Providers from Performing Female Genital Mutilation.* Geneva: WHO. UNAIDS/UNDP/UNFPA/UNICEF/UNHCR/UNIFEM/WHO/FIGO/ICN/IOM/WCPT/WMA/MWIA.

WHO (2011) *Health in the Green Economy: Health Co-benefits of Climate Change Mitigation – Housing Sector.* Geneva: WHO.

WHO (2013) *Comprehensive Mental Health Action Plan 2013–20.* Geneva: WHO. Available at http://apps.who.int/gb/ebwha/pdf_files/WHA66/A66_R8-en.pdf, accessed on 20 April 2014.

WHO Regional Office for Europe (1998) *Health Promotion Evaluation: Recommendations to Policy-Makers. Report of the WHO European Working Group on Health Promotion Evaluation* (document EUR/ICP/IVST 05 01 03). Copenhagen: WHO.

WHO Regional Office for Europe (2012) *Health 2020: A European Policy Framework and Strategy for the 21st Century.* Copenhagen: WHO.

WHO Regional Office for Europe (n.d.) *Healthy Cities.* Copenhagen: WHO. Available at www.euro.who.int/en/health-topics/environment-and-health/urban-health/activities/healthy-cities, accessed on 6 June 2014.

Wikipedia contributors (2012) *Social Networking.* Wikipedia, The Free Encyclopedia. Available at http://en.wikipedia.org/wiki/Social_networking_service, accessed on 13 December 2013.

Wikipedia contributors (2013) *Netmums.* Wikipedia, The Free Encyclopedia. Available at http://en.wikipedia.org/wiki/Netmums, accessed on 13 December 2013.

Wilkinson, R. G. (2005) *The Impact of Inequality: How to Make Sick Societies Healthier.* Abingdon: Routledge.

Wilkinson, R. G. (2007) 'Cut pay to beat poverty.' (Quoted in *Community Practitioner News.*) *Community Practitioner 80*, 12, 6.

Wilkinson, R. G. and Pickett, K. (2009) *The Spirit Level: Why More Equal Societies Almost Always Do Better.* London: Penguin.

Williams, M. and Penman, D. (2011) *Mindfulness.* London: Piatkus.

Wiltshire, S. (2010) *A Select Review of Literature on the Relationship Between Housing and Health.* Edinburgh: Scottish Government Communities Analytical Services. Available at www.scotland.gov.uk/Resource/Doc/1035/0104565.doc, accessed on 3 January 2013.

Windle, K., Francis, J. and Coomber, C. (2011) *Preventing Loneliness and Social Isolation: Interventions and Outcomes. Briefing Paper 39.* London: Social Care Institute for Excellence.

Winkelby, M. A., Rovinson, T. N., Sundquist, J. and Kraemer, H. C. (1999) 'Ethnic variation in cardiovascular disease risk factor among children and young adults: Findings from the third National Health and Nutrition Examination Survey, 1988–1994.' *Journal of the American Medical Association 281*, 11, 1006–1013.

Winters, L., Armitage, M., Stansfield, J., Scott-Samuel, A. and Farrar, A. (2010) *Wellness Services – Evidence Based Review and Examples of Good Practice.* Liverpool: Liverpool Public Health Observatory.

Wolf, O. T. and Buss, C. (2009) *Mental Capital and Wellbeing: Making the Most of Ourselves in the 21st Century. State-of-Science Review: SR-E20. Effect of Chronic Stress on Cognitive Function through Life*. London: Government Office of Science.

Wood, J. (2004) *Rural Health and Healthcare: A North West Perspective. A Public Health Information Report for the North West Public Health Observatory*. Liverpool: North West Public Health Observatory. Available at www.nwpho.org.uk/reports/ ruralhealth.pdf, accessed on 28 July 2013.

Woodhead, C., Rona, R., Iversen, A., MacManus, D., *et al.* (2011) 'Mental health and health service use among post-national service veterans: Results from the 2007 Adult Psychiatric Morbidity Survey of England.' *Psychological Medicine 41*, 363–372.

Woodhead, L. (2009) *'Religion or Belief': Identifying Issues and Priorities. Research Report 48*. London: Equality and Human Rights Commission. Available at www.equalityhumanrights.com/uploaded_files/research/research_report_48__ religion_or_belief.pdf, accessed on 8 December 2013.

Yeandle, S., Bennett, C., Buckner, L., Fry, G. and Price, C. (2012) *Managing Caring and Employment*. Leeds: University of Leeds.

Yeandle, S., Stiell, B. and Buckner, L. (2006) *Ethnic Minority Women and Access to the Labour Market. Synthesis Report*. Sheffield: Centre for Social Inclusion, Sheffield Hallam University.

SUBJECT INDEX

AUTHOR INDEX